Moufida Mahmoudi
Amal Khsiba
Lamine Hamzaoui

# Prevalence of celiac disease in cirrhosis

**Moufida Mahmoudi**
**Amal Khsiba**
**Lamine Hamzaoui**

# Prevalence of celiac disease in cirrhosis

**ScienciaScripts**

This book is a translation from the original published under ISBN 978-620-6-72372-1.

Publisher:
Sciencia Scripts
is a trademark of
Dodo Books Indian Ocean Ltd. and OmniScriptum S.R.L publishing group

120 High Road, East Finchley, London, N2 9ED, United Kingdom
Str. Armeneasca 28/1, office 1, Chisinau MD-2012, Republic of Moldova, Europe
Printed at: see last page
**ISBN: 978-620-8-14309-1**

# PREVALENCE OF CELIAC DISEASE IN CIRRHOSIS AND THE EFFECT OF A GLUTEN-FREE DIET: A PROSPECTIVE STUDY OF 100 CASES

**INTRODUCION**

Celiac disease (CD) is an autoimmune enteropathy induced by ingestion of gluten, a protein derived from wheat, rye and barley, in genetically predisposed individuals (HLA DQ2 or DQ8)[1].

It is a common disease, with a reported prevalence of 1/100 to 1/150000 inhabitants, but is probably underestimated due to the existence of pauci or asymptomatic forms [].

Two peaks in incidence are observed, the first in childhood, the second in adults between the ages of 20 and 40. Diagnosis can take longer, with 20% of adult forms diagnosed after the age of 60[2].

Extradigestive forms reveal the disease in more than 80% of cases [3]. Among the extradigestive manifestations, liver involvement is one of the most frequent.

The involvement of the liver in CD has been widely described in the literature through case series reported over the last four decades. CD has been associated not only with autoimmune hepatopathies such as primary sclerosing cholangitis (PSC), biliary cholangitis (BC), and other autoimmune diseases, but also with a number of other autoimmune diseases.

(CBP) and autoimmune hepatitis (HAI), but also viral hepatitis B and C and non-alcoholic steatohepatitis (NASH), as well as Wilson's disease, cirrhosis and portal hypertension [4].

Swedish epidemiological studies have shown that CD patients have a 2 to 6-fold increased risk of developing liver disease during the course of the disease and an estimated 8-fold increased risk of death from cirrhosis compared with the general population[5]. CD is at least twice as common in cirrhotic patients as in the general population[4].An association between cirrhosis of undetermined aetiology (after excluding viral, metabolic and toxic aetiologies) and CD has also been suggested and described in the literature (case reports) [4, 6, 7]. Early diagnosis of CD in cirrhosis makes it possible to initiate GFR and potentially prevent the morbidity and mortality of both diseases.

Three cases of CD associated with cirrhosis have been reported in the two Gastroenterology departments of Nabeul and Monastir. After reviewing the literature, we conducted this study with the following objectives:

1) Determine the prevalence of CD in cirrhosis

2) Assessing the effect of RSG on liver function

# PATIENTS AND METHODS

## I. Type of study :

This is a prospective, descriptive, observational, bi-centric study of cirrhotic patients treated in the Gastroenterology departments of the Mohamed Taher Maamouri University Hospital Centre (CHU) in Nabeul and the Fattouma Bourguiba CHU in Monastir between 2015 and 2017.

## II. Study population

### Inclusion criteria:

- Patients included in the study were those with cirrhosis, whatever the underlying aetiology, whether or not they had digestive signs.

- The diagnosis of cirrhosis was based on signs of hepatocellular insufficiency and PH: clinico-biological, endoscopic, imaging and progressive.

### Exclusion criteria:

The patients excluded from our study are :
- patients with active bleeding at the time of upper GI endoscopy.

- Patients on anticoagulants with haemostasis disorders.

INR>1.7 and/or platelets <30000elements/mm³.

- Patients with life-limiting malignant tumours

- Patients who have had an organ transplant.

- Patients with chronic renal failure at the dialysis stage.

## III. Methodology :

We included two gastroenterology departments in which gastroenterologists participated in our study. Ideally, they were asked to perform six biopsies (two from the bulb and four from the duodenum) and at least three biopsies. The protocol for our study was displayed in both gastrointestinal endoscopy units. Celiac disease serology was requested in all patients included.

## IV. Data collection :

The data was collected by the doctor in charge of the study, using patient files. Data collection and entry took two years.

Data were collected using a template (Appendix 1): Data on cirrhosis included:

- clinical, biological and morphological data to support the diagnosis of cirrhosis:

➢ clinical signs of hepatocellular failure and PH

➢ biological data, in particular blood count and formula, prothrombin level, INR, transaminases, total and conjugated bilirubin, protein electrophoresis.

➢ morphological data: signs of PH on abdominal ultrasound (dilatation of the portal trunk, collateral venous circulation, splenomegaly and ascites) with liver dysmorphia and on endoscopy (oesophageal varices, gastric varices and hypertensive gastropathy)

- how cirrhosis develops and how long it lasts

- severity of cirrhosis: Child-Pugh score and MELD score were calculated for all patients at inclusion.

- Etiological assessment of cirrhosis :

➢ B and C viral serologies

➢ immunological work-up; antinuclear antibodies, anti-smooth muscle antibodies, anti-LKM1 antibodies, anti-mitochondrial antibodies

➢ weight measurement of immunoglobulins

➢ lipid levels, blood sugar levels

➢ Abdominal Doppler ultrasound

➢ The balance sheet copper balance, alpha1-antitrypsin, the ferritinemia, transferrin saturation coefficient.

- Complications that have occurred during the course of cirrhosis and their treatment:

➢ oedemato-ascitic decompensation

➢ digestive haemorrhage

➤ hepatic encephalopathy
➤ spontaneous infection of ascites fluid
➤ Hepatorenal syndrome

➤ refractory ascites.

- Etiological treatment of cirrhosis :

➤ Antiviral treatment
➤ Ursodeoxycholic acid

➤ D-Penicillamine
➤ Azathioprine.
Data on celiac disease included:
- Serological data :

Measurement of anti-TTG and anti-EMA antibodies.

Anti-gliadin antibodies are less sensitive and less specific, so they were not used in our study.
A weighted IgA assay was performed in the event of an undetectable level of anti-TTG IgA.

- Endoscopic data :

The endoscopic appearance of the duodenum at oeso-gastroduodenal endoscopy: crenellated appearance of the duodenal folds, rarefaction of the duodenal folds, reduced valvular folding, mosaic appearance, erosive or ulcerated duodenitis, duodenal lymphangiectasia.
- Histological data: the result of the duodenal biopsy.
For patients with celiac disease, we specified :
- the interval between the diagnosis of cirrhosis and that of coeliac disease

- symptoms associated with coeliac disease

- whether or not the biology shows malabsorption syndrome

- compliance with the gluten-free diet.

Patients with cirrhosis and MC were followed until the end of August 2017.

**V.Monitoring procedures :**

- Monitoring was carried out once a month during the first trimester, then once a trimester for a year, and thereafter according to both liver and intestinal damage.
- Monitoring was based on :

➤ Clinical monitoring: looking for weight gain and the disappearance or improvement of symptoms and clinical signs, especially in the first 3 months.
➤ Biological monitoring: with an analysis of the blood count and formula, serum ferritin, liver function tests, renal function tests, blood albumin and prothrombin levels.
➤ Serological monitoring: at one year, to look for any negativation of autoantibodies.

➤ Histological monitoring: at least one year later, looking for villous regrowth and a reduction in intra-epithelial lymphocytosis for intestinal involvement.
➤ Bone densitometry monitoring was indicated after one year of GSR when the initial results were pathological.
➤ Ultrasound monitoring was recommended every 6 months.


**VI.  Statistical analysis :**

Data were coded and entered on an SPSS 21.0 computer, with qualitative variables described by proportions and quantitative variables by means and standard deviation. The Chi2 test was used for univariate analysis with a significance level of 5%.

**VII. Bibliographic research**


We consulted a large number of scientific articles in the database of various websites:

Pubmed: http://www.ncbi.nih.gov/pumed Science direct : http://www.sicencedirect.com Google scholar: http://www.scholargoogle.com Articles and journals were searched in both French and English using key words such as celiac disease, cirrhosis and histology.

We also consulted the various theses published on websites (the last search was carried out in April 2017).

Bibliography and reference management were carried out using EndNote X7 software.

## VIII. Ethical considerations :

Medical confidentiality was respected for all observations concerning patient identity and medical data. The content and condition of the files were respected.

We had no conflicts of interest to declare.

## IX. Operational definitions :

### IX .1. Positive diagnosis of cirrhosis :

The diagnosis of cirrhosis was based on a combination of clinical, biological, morphological and endoscopic evidence. Liver biopsy was requested only when the diagnosis was uncertain.

### IX.2. Prognostic scores :

**IX.2.a**  Child-Pugh score:

This is a prognostic score for cirrhosis. This assessment is based on five parameters: bilirubin, albumin, prothrombin time (PT), ascites and encephalopathy (appendix 2).

**IX.2.b**  MELD score: (model for end-stage liver disease)

The MELD score is used to assess and predict mortality in the short and medium term; three to twelve months following surgery such as TIPS or major surgery in patients with cirrhosis.

The MELD score can also be used to predict mortality in a number of clinical situations such as alcoholic hepatitis, type 2 hepatorenal syndrome, sepsis in cirrhosis, acute liver failure and ruptured oesophageal varices.

This score comprises four variables: serum total bilirubin (Tb) concentration, serum creatinine, INR and cause of cirrhosis (Appendix 3).


**IX.3.** Positive diagnosis of celiac disease :

IX.3.a Celiac disease serology :

A value for anti-EMA antibodies (enzyme-linked immunosorbent assay) is considered positive if it is ≥ 10 IU/mL, and a level of anti-TTG antibodies (indirect immunofluorescence assay) is considered positive if it is ≥ 20 IU/mL.

IX.3.b Histological diagnosis of celiac disease :


- Duodenal biopsies are fixed in a 10% formalin solution and analysed by experienced pathologists.
- They were not informed about our study.

- Histological abnormalities are classified according to the Marsh-Oberhuber stage (Appendix 4).

Note that the most severe degree of atrophy is taken into account when there are two degrees of atrophy on the biopsies.

The diagnosis of CD is accepted when celiac serology is positive with duodenal villous atrophy, i.e. Marsh-Oberhuber stage III[6] (appendix 5).

## A. Socio-demographic and clinical characteristics of patients

### 1) Socio-demographic characteristics :

One hundred patients were included in our study, 55 men and 45 women (sex ratio 1.22). The mean age of our patients was 57 years (range 18-94 years), and most were over 40 years of age (89%). Figure 1 shows the distribution of patients by age.

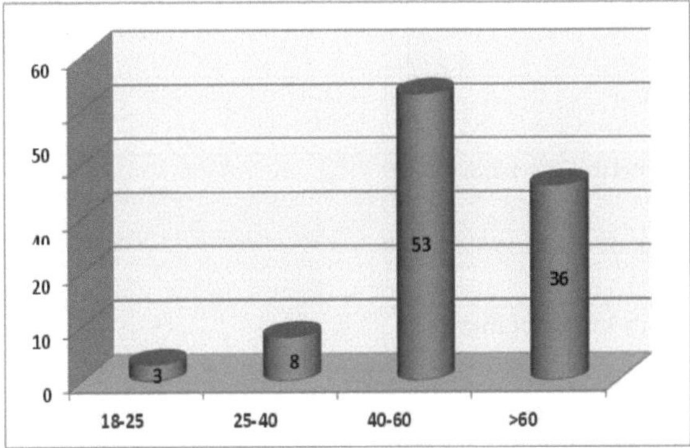


**Figure 1**: Distribution of patients by age group.

The average follow-up of our patients for cirrhosis was 5.6 years (2-15 years). A history of autoimmune diseases was noted in 13% of cases. Chronic alcoholism was noted in 5% of cases. Socio-demographic and patient characteristics are shown in Table 1.

**Table 1:** Socio-demographic and clinical characteristics of patients

| variables | N (=100) |
|---|---|
| Age (years) :<br>-<under 40<br>->40 years | 11<br>89 |
| Sex ratio (M/F) | 1,22 |
| Active smoking | 16 |
| Chronic alcoholism | 5 |
| Type 2 diabetes | 6 |
| HTA | 28 |
| Dysmetabolic syndrome | 29 |
| Hepatitis risk factors | 69 |
| Family history of liver disease chronicle | 6 |
| Autoimmune diseases<br>Autoimmune thyroiditis<br>Type 1 diabetes<br>Vitiligo | <br>9<br>3<br>1 |

## 2) Characteristics of cirrhosis :

In our series, the diagnosis of cirrhosis was made on the basis of clinical, biological, endoscopic and evolutionary evidence. Histological analysis of the liver was performed in 7% of cases. Cryptogenic cirrhosis was the most frequent, occurring in 39% of cases. The other causes of cirrhosis are shown in Figure 2.

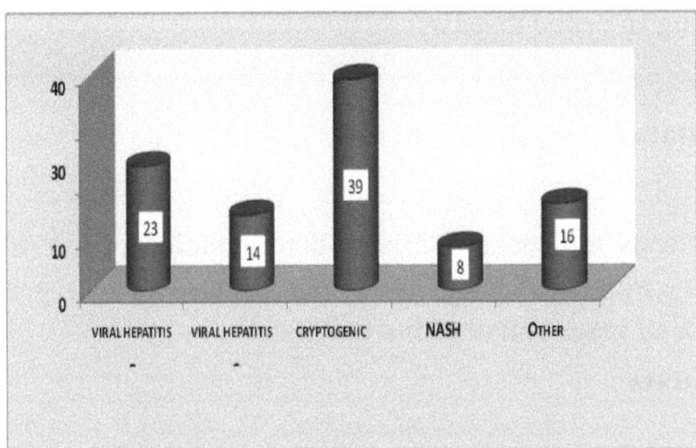


**Figure 2:**Aetiologies of cirrhosis

At the time of inclusion, 91% of patients had decompensated cirrhosis. The characteristics of cirrhosis are shown in Table 2.

**Table 2**: Characteristics of cirrhosis

| | Viral hepatitis B | Viral hepatitis C | Cryptogenic | NASH | Other |
|---|---|---|---|---|---|
| Score Child -pugh A B C | 6 14 3 | 10 3 1 | 12 23 4 | 6 2 0 | 7 8 1 |
| MELD score - ≤12 - > 12 | 8 15 | 9 15 | 20 19 | 5 3 | 8 8 |
| Etiological treatment Yes No | 17 6 | 0 14 | 0 39 | 0 8 | 10 6 |
| Upper GI haemorrhage secondary to PH | 3 | 2 | 13 | 2 | 3 |
| Oedema decompensation ascitic | 15 | 7 | 23 | 1 | 6 |
| Spontaneous fluid infection ascites | 9 | 0 | 3 | 0 | 0 |
| Hepatic encephalopathy | 3 | 1 | 6 | 2 | 0 |
| Hepatorenal syndrome | 0 | 0 | 2 | 0 | 4 |
| Hydrothorax | 1 | 0 | 3 | 0 | 1 |

**B.  Data relating to celiac disease :**

**1) Serological data :**

Immunological tests for coeliac disease (determination of anti-EMA and anti-TTG antibodies) were carried out in all our patients. It was positive for both antibodies in 4% of cases and negative in 86%.

**2) Endoscopic data :**

All our patients underwent oesogastroduodenal endoscopy (EOGD) with duodeno-jejunal biopsies. The endoscopic findings are shown in Table 3.

**Table 3:** The different endoscopic aspects of the duodenum

| Endoscopic aspects duodenum | Number of cases | Percentage (%) |
|---|---|---|
| Normal | 86 | 86% |
| Reduction in duodenal folding | 1 | 1% |
| Mosaic appearance | 4 | 4% |
| Crenellated appearance of the folds | 1 | 1% |
| Ulcerative duodenitis | 4 | 4% |
| Congestive duodenitis | 2 | 2% |
| Aspect of lymphangiectasia | 2 | 2% |

**3) Histological data :**

Data from duodenal biopsies taken during EOGD are summarised in Table 4.

**Table 4: Histological data from duodenal biopsies**

| Biopsy results duodenal | Number of cases | Percentage (%) |
|---|---|---|
| Normal | 84 | 84% |
| Villi atrophy | 4 | 4% |
| Hyper lymphocytosis intraepithelial | 3 | 3% |
| Inflammatory duodenitis | 9 | 9% |

## C. Prevalence of coeliac disease in our study:

Only one patient    had positive CD serology with villous atrophy on duodenal biopsy, confirming the diagnosis of CD. Thus, the prevalence of CD in cirrhotic patients in our study is 1%. The aetiology of cirrhosis in this patient was cryptogenic. The prevalence of CD in cryptogenic cirrhosis is 2.5%.

## D. Analysis of comments :

In what follows, we report the case of a patient with cirrhosis and CD detected by our study, as well as the three cases of CD and cirrhosis collected in the gastroenterology departments of Nabeul and Monastir.

**1) First observation:**

Patient M.S, aged 41, with a history of iron-deficiency anaemia, who had been started on martial therapy without exploration, consulted his doctor with an anaemic syndrome consisting of asthenia and dizziness associated with abdominal distension that had been evolving for a fortnight prior to admission. Clinical examination revealed thinness (BMI = $18.7\text{kg/m}^2$), paleness of the conjunctiva and trophic disorders of the skin and mucosa (hypoplasia of the dental enamel with dry, thinning hair). Neurological examination was normal.

Abdominal examination revealed sloping dullness of the flanks, CVC and SMG. The initial biological examination showed :

-A malabsorption syndrome with severe anaemia (Hb = 3g/dl) hypochromic (CCMH = 27g/dl) microcytic (VGM = 73fL), iron deficiency (ferritinaemia at 4 µg/L), hypocholesterolaemia at 2mmol/L (N: 3.7 to 6.50), hypo-triglyceridaemia at 0.5 mmol/L (N: 0.6 to 1.7) and hypo albuminaemia at 23 g/L.

- Corrected serum calcium was normal.

- Hepatic cytolysis: ASAT 2N and ALAT 1.5N.

- Coagulation times were normal.

-The ascites was transudative and poor in cells.

Given this biological picture, which combined hypocholesterolaemia with iron-deficiency anaemia and hypoalbuminemia, malabsorption was suspected.

Further questioning revealed long-standing digestive disorders with alternating normal transit and intermittent diarrhoea, and anaemic episodes resistant to martial therapy. An upper gastrointestinal endoscopy showed small oesophageal varices (grade 1) and moderate hypertensive gastritis with crenellated duodenal folds (image 1).

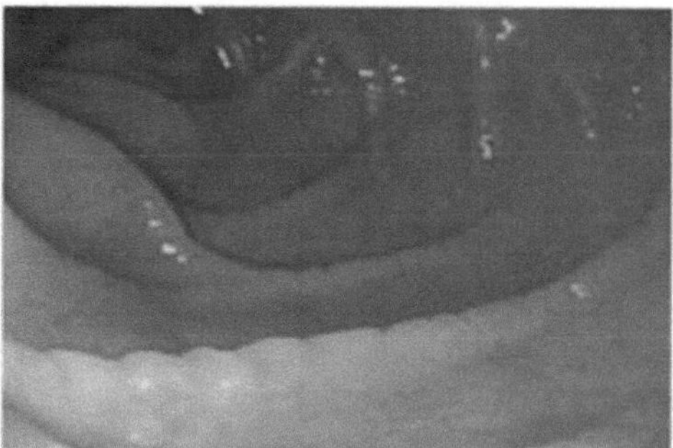

**Image 1**: crenellated appearance of the duodenal folds

Pathological examination revealed total villous atrophy and crypt hyperplasia with epithelial lymphocytosis (image 2).

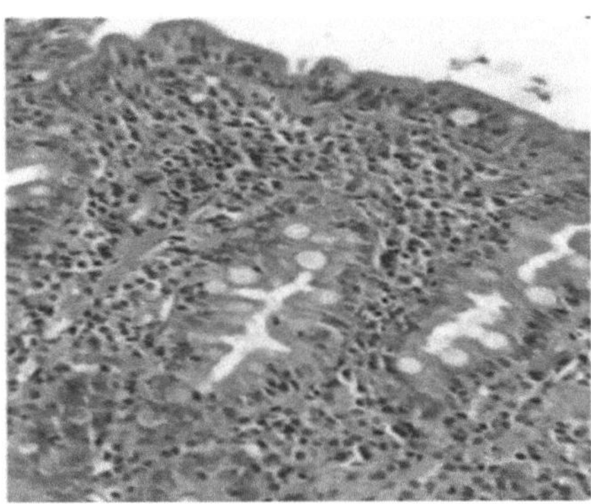

**Image 2:** Histological aspect of a duodenal biopsy showing villous atrophy with crypt hyperplasia

IgA anti-TTG and anti-EMA antibodies were positive. The diagnosis of CD was accepted.

As part of the aetiological work-up for PH, an abdominal ultrasound scan showed hepatic dysmorphia, SMG and CVC with a moderate amount of peritoneal effusion.

The diagnosis of cirrhosis was based on clinico-biological, radiological and endoscopic evidence of PH and hepatocellular failure. She was classified as Child -Pugh B7.

The aetiological work-up for cirrhosis, including viral serology (B and C), immunological work-up and copper work-up, was negative.

The patient was started on RSG. The outcome was favourable, with resolution of ascites on diuretic treatment, resolution of digestive symptoms and significant villous regrowth on duodenal biopsies taken 1 year later.

As regards liver function, an improvement in the Child-Pugh score was noted: A5 at 1 year. The patient did not present any decompensation of cirrhosis after a follow-up of 3 years. Table 5 summarises the patient's laboratory investigations.

Table 5: Results of biological tests for the first observation

| Parameters | Results |
|---|---|
| Leukocytes Platelets<br>Prothrombin rate Albuminemia<br>Bt ASAT ALAT<br>Alkaline phosphatases GGT<br>Vitamin B12<br>Anti Intrinsic Factor Ac Anti<br>Parietal Cell Ac | 2500 (N : 4-10 elm/mm³)<br>88000 (N : 150-400 × 10³)<br>74% (N: 75-100 %)<br>23(<17µmol/l)<br>23 (N: 35-50 g/L)<br>81 IU/L (N: 5-45 IU/L)<br>70 IU/L (N: 5-45 IU/L)<br>314 IU/L (N: 98-279 IU/L)<br>151 UI/L (N: 11-50 UI/L)<br>350 (130 and 800 ng / l) Negative<br>Negative |
| Anti-TTG Ac Anti-EMA Ac | Positive Positive |

## 2) Second observation:

Mr L.A, aged 39, with no particular pathological history, was admitted for investigation of transit disorders of the alternating diarrhoea-constipation type with epigastric abdominal pain that had been evolving for 3 months in a context of deteriorating general condition.

On physical examination, the patient's general condition showed little change, with a body mass index (BMI) of 24.8 kg/m². The patient had pale skin and mucous membranes; he was apyretic. Abdominal examination showed SMG.

The laboratory work-up revealed pancytopenia: leukopenia (white blood cells were $1.9 × 10^3$ el/mm³), iron-deficiency microcytic hypochromic anaemia (6.3g/dL) and thrombocytopenia ($110 × 10^3$ el/L).

Hepatic cytolysis was observed, with a predominance of ASAT at 1.5 times normal: 60 IU/L (N < 40 IU/L) and ALAT at 1.35 times normal: 54 IU/L (N < 40 IU/L).

Cholestasis tests, prothrombin levels (PT), lipid and renal profiles, albumin levels, blood glucose and blood calcium levels were all normal.

Viral serologies (B and C) and immunological tests (anti-nuclear Ac, anti-smooth muscle Ac and anti-LKM1 Ac) were negative, with a normal Ig weight assay. Ophthalmic examination showed no pericorneal ring.

The copper profile and alpha 1 antitrypsin assay were normal. Anti-EMA and anti-TTG antibodies were positive. Abdominal ultrasound showed an enlarged liver with normal echostructure, regular contours and splenomegaly. The portal trunk and splenic vein were of normal calibre. Upper gastrointestinal endoscopy revealed large oesophageal varices (grade II) with a mosaic appearance of the duodenal mucosa.

Duodenal biopsy showed total villous atrophy (image 3) consistent with celiac disease without histological signs of malignancy.

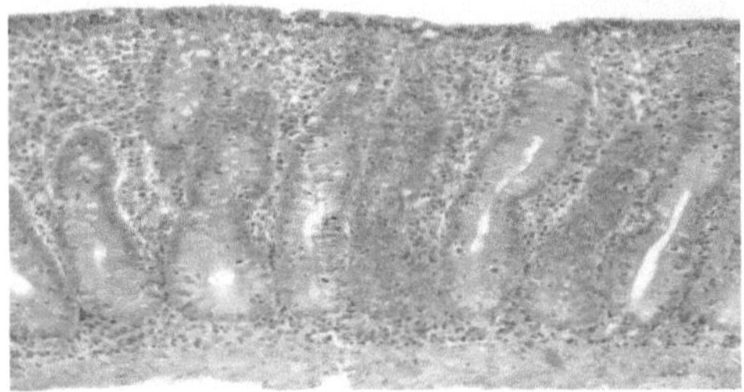

**Image 3**: Duodenal biopsy showing total villous atrophy
Colonoscopy was also normal.

Transparietal liver biopsy (TPL) showed chronic liver disease at the stage of minimal cirrhosis classified as A1F4 according to Metavir (image 4).

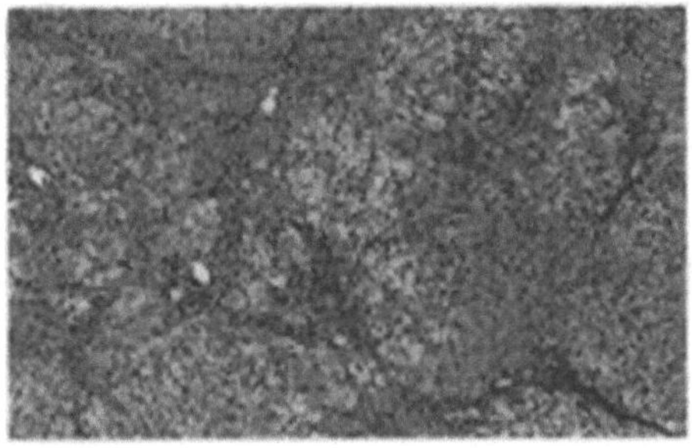

**Image 4:**liver biopsy showing liver disease at cirrhosis stage

On the basis of these clinical and paraclinical data, the diagnosis was cryptogenic cirrhosis associated with CD. The cirrhosis was classified as Child-Pugh A5.The patient was put on RSG with good compliance. Vitamin supplementation and martial therapy were prescribed. A clinical check-up at 3 months showed a weight gain of 2 kg. At one year, specific antibodies had become negative and villous atrophy had regressed on duodenal biopsy.

Biologically, hepatic cytolysis had regressed; ALT: 50IU/l (1.1N), ASAT: 45IU/l (N), and albumin and prothrombin levels were stable (normal). A follow-up PBH, with the patient's agreement, was planned in order to assess the effect of RSG on the regression of fibrosis.

The results of the laboratory tests are shown in Table 6.

**Table 6:** Results of biological investigations for the second observation

| Parameters | Results |
|---|---|
| Leukocytes Haemoglobin VGM | 1.9 × 103/L (N: 4-10 × 103/L) |
| CCMH | 6.3 g/dL (N: 115-160) |
| Inserts | 55 fl (N: 84-96) |
| Sedimentation rate Prothrombin | 27 % (N : 31-36) |
| rate Albuminemia Protidemia | 110 ×103/L (N: 150-400 × 103) |
| Blood glucose Cholesterol Total | 17 mm (N < 20 mm) |
| bilirubin ASAT | 90 % (N : 75-100 %) |
| ALAT | 38 (N: 35-50 g/L) |
| Alkaline phosphatases GGT | 70 (N: 60-80 g/L) |
| Serum calcium Creatinine Serum | 4.9 mmol/L (N: 3.33-6.10 |
| iron Ferritinemia HBs antigen | mmol/L) |
| Anti-HVC antibodies Anti-TTG | 2.1 mmol/L (N: 3.47-6.45 |
| antibodies Anti-EMA antibodies | mmol/L) |
| Anti-nuclear antibodies Anti- | 8 mol/L (N: 1-12mol/L) |
| smooth muscle antibodies Anti- | 54 IU/L (N: 5-45 IU/L) |
| mitochondria antibodies | 60 IU/L (N: 5-45 IU/L) |
| Anti-KLM1 antibodies | 61 UI/L (N: 98-279 UI/L) |
| | 40 UI/L (N: 11-50 UI/L) |
| | 1.88 mmol/L (N: 2.1-2.6 mmol/L) |
| | 61 µmol/L (N: 53-97 µmol/L) |
| | 3.30 mmol/L (N:2.49-7.49 |
| | mmol/L) |
| | 2.13 µg/L (N: 15-150 µg/L) |
| | Negative Negative Positive |
| | Positive Negative Negative |
| | Negative Negative |

VGM: mean corpuscular volume; CCMH: mean corpuscular haemoglobin concentration; LDH: lactate dehydrogenase

## 3) Comment 3:

Patient H.M.J, aged 20, from a consanguineous marriage (1ᵉʳ degree), was admitted for investigation of cholestatic icterus with right hypochondrial pain. Questioning revealed a family history of death in the neonatal period and during childhood of a brother and two cousins with jaundice of unspecified aetiology. He had no particular personal pathological history. The patient smoked 4 times a day and had no history of alcohol consumption or hepatitis risk factors.

Symptoms had been present for 1 month and began with abdominal pain, followed by the onset of mucocutaneous jaundice with dark urine and no discolouration of the stools, evolving in a context of weight loss that had not been quantified.On clinical examination, the patient was apyretic and lean (BMI = 17kg/m²) with mucocutaneous jaundice and no signs of hepatocellular failure. Haemodynamic and respiratory constants were normal. The neurological examination was unremarkable. Abdominal examination showed slight tenderness of the right hypochondrium and MGS with no hepatomegaly, CVC or ascites. Dermatological examination revealed papular and scaly lesions on the trunk, both forearms and both lower limbs, with pigmentation of the palms and soles (image 5).

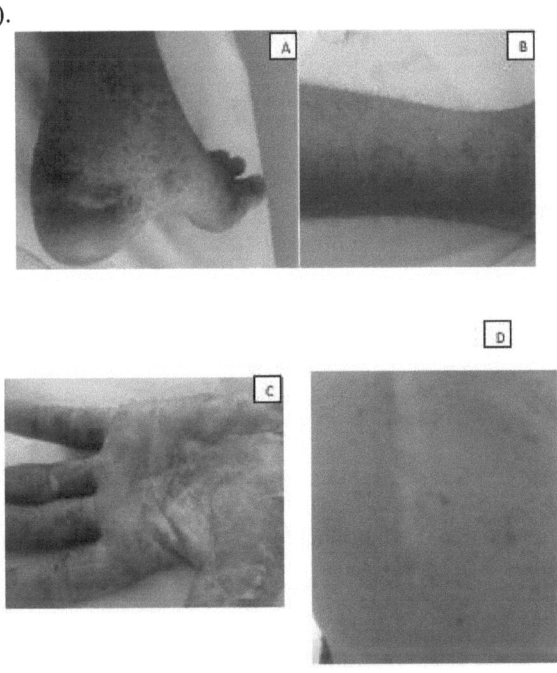

**Image 5:** Squames and bullae on extremities (A-B), pigmentation on palms and feet (A-C), erythematous lesions on trunk and legs (B, D).

The biological work-up showed :

- A normal blood count and formula without hyper eosinophilia.

- Hepatic cytolysis, with ALT predominating (55 times normal) and ASAT 95 times normal.

- Jaundiced hepatic cholestasis: alkaline phosphatases at 1.5 N, GGT at 2 N, Bt at 540 µmol/l (N < 17 µmol/l), predominantly conjugated at 401 µmol/l.

- Hepatocellular failure: prothrombin level 40%, INR 1.69, hypo albuminemia 27 g/L and hypocholesterolemia 2 mmol/L.

Abdominal ultrasound showed :

➢ A normal liver,

➢ A homogeneous SMG,

➢ A thickened, undistended gallbladder with alithiasis,

➢ Non-dilated intra- and extra-hepatic bile ducts. The oeso-gastro-duodenal endoscopy had noted :
➢ The absence of oesophageal and/or gastric varices

➢ Erosive fundic gastritis

➢ Congestive antrhitis

This was a case of severe acute hepatitis in a 20-year-old patient with a family history of unlabelled jaundice.

• An exhaustive aetiological work-up was carried out:

➢ Drug and toxic causes ruled out on examination

➢ Negative A / B / C / E viral serologies

➢ The ophthalmological examination showed the presence of a Kayser-Fleischer ring (bilateral).

☐ Given the following arguments :

• Young age

• Family history of jaundice

• The picture of acute hepatitis

• The presence of a bilateral Kayser-Fleischer ring led to the diagnosis of Wilson's disease.

A copper assessment was carried out and treatment with D-Penicillamine was started before the results of the assessment were available. A specialist neurological examination showed an abolition of achilles reflexes and axonal sensory-motor polyneuropathy in the four proximal and distal limbs, with greater severity in the two lower limbs on electromyography. On brain MRI, the hypothalamic-pituitary axis appeared normal, with a bipallidal T1 hyper signal suggestive of cerebral involvement in Wilson's disease.

Cardiac ultrasound was normal.

The patient also attended a specialist dermatology consultation, where various diagnoses were suggested: porphyria, toxidermia, etc. Skin biopsies were taken, but were non-specific (scarring lesions). The patient was put on topical treatment (salicylated petroleum jelly / antiseptic solution / eosin treatments).

➤ Non-literate viral hepatitis serologies: cytomegalovirus (CMV), HSV1 and 2 were negative. Epstein-Barr virus (EBV) serology was consistent with a long-standing infection. HIV serology was negative.
➤ Non-viral infectious causes: syphilitic serology, Vidal serology = negative
➤ Antinuclear, anti-smooth muscle, anti-LKM1 and anti-mitochondrial antibodies = negative.

The weighted Ig assay showed IgM at 1.11 g/l (N = 0.55-1.96 g/l), IgA at 1.55 g/l (N = 0.77-2.48) and normal IgG.

➤ Measurement of serum ferritin, ceruloplasmin, cupraemia, cupruria, α1 antitrypsin = normal.
➤ Porphyria work-up = normal

The patient was initially kept on D-Penicillamine with vitamin K supplementation. Clinically, there was a disappearance of skin lesions and an initial improvement in jaundice without disappearance.

Biological changes are shown in Table 7.

Table 7: Changes in biological check-up

| Date: 2014 Balance sheet | 23 August | 31 August | September | December |
|---|---|---|---|---|
| ASAT | 42 N | 26 N | 11 N | 2 N |
| ALAT | 25 N | 19 N | 4 N | 7 N |
| Bil T/C | 510/497 | 496/400 | 426/390 | 206/127 |
| PAL | 1,25 N | 1,5 N | 1,5 N | 5 N |
| GGT | normal | 1,5 N | normal | 6 N |
| TP | 26% | 39% | 58% | 35% |

Transparietal PBH, performed when the PT was 58%, showed : Chronic active liver disease at the stage of cirrhosis, with lesions such as ballooning and hepatocyte clarification, microvacuolar steatosis, signs of cholestasis and an inflammatory infiltrate of neutrophils. There was no iron overload and Perls staining was negative (image 6). This appearance could suggest steatohepatitis, mitochondrial cytopathy or Wilson's disease.  However, rhodanine stainingwas negativeand hepatic copper levels were normal (0.45µmol/g dry tissue).

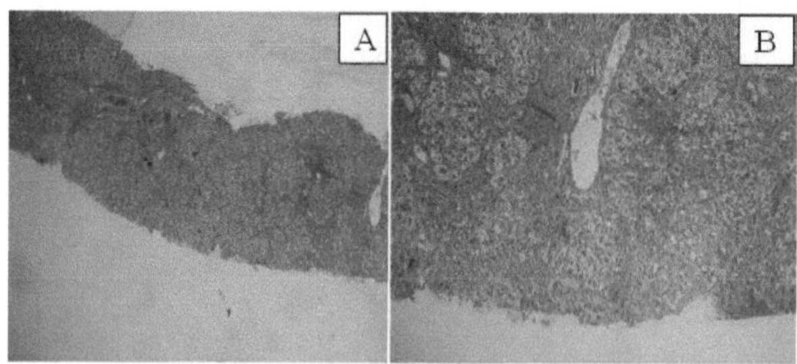

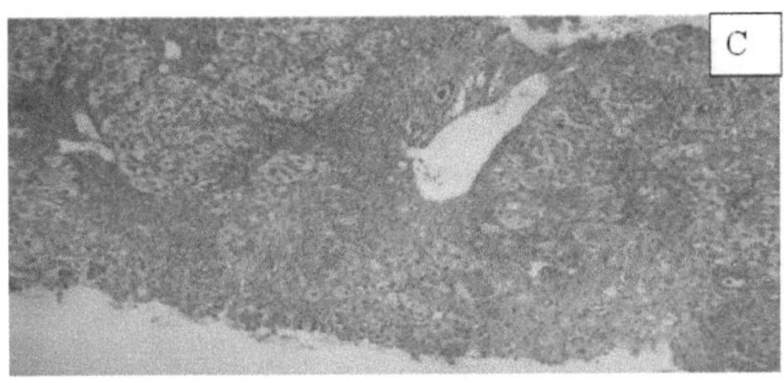

**Image 6:** Histological sections of liver biopsy showing: chronic active liver disease at cirrhosis stage (A+B), microvacuolar steatosis and an inflammatory infiltrate of neutrophils(C)

➤ Mitochondrial cytopathy, but involvement of the central and peripheral nervous systems was subclinical and liver involvement was inaugural.

➤ Familial hypermanganesemia: normal manganese levels

➤ Celiac disease

• Upper gastrointestinal endoscopy was repeated and revealed congestive, ulcerated antral gastritis with a mosaic-like appearance of the duodenal mucosa.

• Duodenal biopsies: pathological examination showed total villous atrophy with intraepithelial hyperlymphocytosis (>40%) and a lymphoplasmacytic inflammatory infiltrate.

• CD serology was positive f o r  anti-TTG and anti-EMA antibodies.

• We reported a case of severe acute hepatitis in a liver with cryptogenic chronic liver disease revealing CD.

The patient was put on RSG, which was poorly monitored. He was rehospitalised one month later with oedemato-ascitic decompensation, ascites fluid infection and stage II hepatic encephalopathy. He was started on antibiotics.

The cirrhosis was classified as Child-Pugh C, MELD 33 Abdominal CT showed:
☐ Retroperitoneal nodular contrast (D3?)

☐ Multiple homogeneous mesenteric adenomegalia

☐ Jejunization of the ileal intestines

☐ Permeability of digestive vessels

Lymphoma was suspected. Jejunoscopy showed multiple duodenal ulcers with necrotic centres (image 7). Jejunal biopsies showed ulcerated duodenojejunitis.

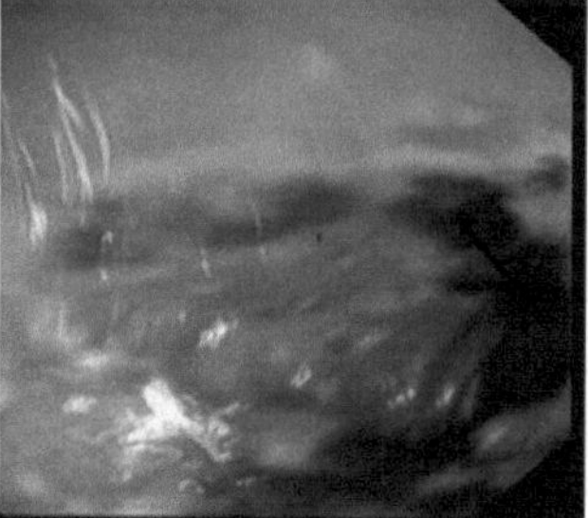

**Image7** : Endoscopic appearance of ulcerated and necrotic jejunitis
After 7 months' follow-up, the patient died of Stenotrophomonas Maltofilia (BGN) septicaemia.Table 8 summarises the patient's laboratory investigations.

**Table 8**: Results of biological investigations in the third observation

| Parameter | Results |
|---|---|
| Leukocytes Haemoglobin Prothrombin rate Albuminemia Bt Bc ASAT ALAT Alkaline phosphatases GGT Serum serum HBS antigen Anti-HVC antibodies HSV1 and 2 serology CMV serology HIV serology EBV serology | 12300 (N: 4-10 × 10³/L) 13,4 (N : 115-160) 40% (N: 75-100 %) 27 (N: 35-50 g/L) 540 μmol/l (<17μmol/l) 401 μmol/l (<17μmol/l) 4275 IU/L (N: 5-45 IU/L) 2475 IU/L (N: 5-45 IU/L) 418 IU/L (N: 98-279 IU/L) 100 UI/L (N: 11-50 UI/L) 859μg /L (30 - 300 μg /L) Negative Negative Negative Negative Negative Negative Old immunity |
| Anti-TTG antibodies Anti-EMA antibodies Ceruloplasmin Cupraemia Cupruria α 1 antitrypsin Urinary porphyrin Faecal porphyrin | Positive Positive 0.27 g/L (0.15-0.6) 0.91mg/L (0.6-1.4mg/l) 83 μg/24h(<100 μg /24h) 2.84g/L (0.9 -2g/l) 15.3 nmol/L (<30) 13nmol/g stool (<200) |

## 4) Observation 4:

Patient H.H, aged 48, with no notable pathological history, was admitted for investigation of abdominal distension that had been evolving for three weeks prior to admission.

Careful questioning revealed a history of gluten intolerance diagnosed at the age of 18, but the patient was not being monitored and was not on a GFD.

The clinical examination showed that the patient was in average general condition, with a BMI of 19.47 kg/m² and oedema of the lower limbs. The neurological examination was unremarkable. Abdominal examination revealed moderate ascites and CVC.

At the biology test, the patient had:

• microcytic hypochromic anaemia at 9g/dl, iron deficiency (serum ferritin at 27 µg/l).
• Hepatic cytolysis: ALT 1.6 N, ASAT 1.12 N, without cholestasis.
• The prothrombin rate was lowered to 63%.
• Biological malabsorption syndrome: iron deficiency anaemia, hypocholesterolaemia and hypo albuminaemia

Abdominal ultrasound showed a dysmorphic liver with heterogeneous echostructure, signs of PH, SMG and moderate ascites, with portal vein thrombosis.

Upper gastrointestinal endoscopy revealed large oesophageal varices (grade II) with a congestive appearance of the duodenal mucosa.

Duodenal biopsy revealed total villous atrophy consistent with CD without histological signs of malignancy.

CD serology was positive for anti-EMA and anti-TTG antibodies.

The diagnosis was oedemato-ascitic decompensated cirrhosis associated with CD and portal vein thrombosis. The cirrhosis was classified as Child-Pugh B8.

In the aetiological work-up for cirrhosis, the B and C viral serologies and the immunological work-up were negative.

The copper balance and alpha 1 antitrypsin assay were normal.

The thrombophilia work-up revealed a reduction in protein C: 55%(VN: 70-120%) and protein S: 30%(VN: 65-140%). The patient was put on RSG, a martial treatment with vitamin supplementation. An anticoagulant treatment was prescribed after eradication of the oesophageal varices by elastic ligation.

An abdominal angioscan, carried out after 6 months of anticoagulant treatment, noted the persistence of portal trunk thrombosis. The patient was poorly compliant with the GVSR, with a positive CD serology test and persistent total villous atrophy on histological examination.

After 9 months, the patient suffered a second oedemato-ascitic decompensation requiring diuretic treatment, with good progression. The cirrhosis was classified as Child-Pugh B9. Table 9 summarises the patient's laboratory investigations.

**Table 9:** Results of biological investigations for the fourth observation

| Parameters | Results |
|---|---|
| Leukocytes Haemoglobin Platelets<br>VGM<br>Prothrombin levels Albumin levels<br>Blood glucose levels<br>Bt ASAT ALAT<br>Alkaline phosphatases GGT<br>Creatinine Anti-TTG mAb Anti-EMA mAb<br>Anti-nuclear antibodies | 4500 (N: 4-10 × 10³/L)<br>90 (N : 115-160)<br>141000 (N : 150-400 × 10³)<br>71fl (N: 84-96)<br>63% (N : 75-100 %)<br>32(<17µmol/l)<br>4.8mmol/L (N: 3.33-6.10 mmol/L)<br>19 (N: 35-50 g/L)<br>64UI/L (N: 5-45 UI/L)<br>45 IU/L (N: 5-45 IU/L)<br>114 IU/L (N: 98-279 IU/L)<br>35 IU/L (N: 11-50 IU/L)<br>72µmol/L (N: 53-97 µmol/L)<br>Positive<br>Positive Negative |
| Anti-smooth muscle antibody<br>Anti-mitochondria antibody Anti-KLM1 antibody<br>B/C viral serology | Negative Negative Negative<br>Negative |

Table 10 summarises the clinical, biological and evolutionary data for the four cases.

**Table10**: Comparative table of the four cases and assessment of liver function before and after the gluten-free diet

| Patients | Our patient | | Cases already reported | | | | | |
|---|---|---|---|---|---|---|---|---|
| | Observation 1 | | Observation 2 | | Observation 3 | | Observation 4 | |
| Gender | Male | | Male | | Male | | Male | |
| Age | 41 | | 39 | | 20 | | 48 | |
| Causes of cirrhosis | Cryptogenic | | Cryptogenic | | Cryptogenic | | Cryptogenic | |
| Associated renal disease | No | | No | | No | | No | |
| Pre-Post RSG | Pré | Post | Pré | Post | Pré | Post | Pré | Post |
| Ac Anti EMA | + | - | + | - | + | | + | + |
| Anti TTG Ac | + | - | + | - | + | | + | + |
| Marsh Stadium | IIIc | II | IIIc | IIIc | IIIc | | IIIc | IIIc |
| BMI | 18,7 | 21,6 | 24,8 | 25,85 | 16,9 | | 19,74 | 21,5 |
| BT | 20 | 11 | 10 | 15 | 592 | | 67 | 78 |
| ASAT | 81 | 55 | 54 | 45 | 420 | | 45 | 60 |
| ALAT | 70 | 62 | 60 | 50 | 2200 | | 64 | 87 |
| TP | 74% | 77% | 90% | 87% | 52% | | 63% | 50% |
| Albumin | 23 | 36 | 38 | 37 | 27,5 | | 29 | 25 |
| Alkaline phosphatase | 314 | 211 | 61 | 75 | 418,5 | | 114 | 234 |
| INR | 1,4 | 1,52 | 1,6 | 1,54 | 1,69 | | 1,59 | 1,8 |
| Creatinemia | 57 | 53 | 65 | 58 | 65 | | 43 | 82 |
| Score Child | B7 | A5 | A5 | A5 | C | | B8 | B9 |
| Meld score | 12 | 11 | 12 | 11 | 26 | | 17 | 19 |
| Complications: | | | | | | | | |
| Digestive haemorrhage | 0 | 0 | 0 | 0 | 0 | | + | 0 |
| Hepatorenal syndrome | 0 | 0 | 0 | 0 | 0 | | 0 | 0 |
| Hepatic encephalopathy | 0 | 0 | 0 | 0 | + | | 0 | 0 |
| DOA | + | 0 | 0 | 0 | + | | + | 0 |
| Deaths | No | | No | | Yes | | No | |

# DISCUSSION

Our study included 100 patients, mean age 57 [18; 94], with cirrhosis of various aetiologies who underwent CD serology associated with duodenal biopsy. The aim of this study was to determine the prevalence of CD in cirrhotic patients and to evaluate the effect of GSR on liver function in cases of associated CD. At the end of the study, the prevalence of CD in cirrhosis was estimated at 1% across all aetiologies and 2.5% in cryptogenic cirrhosis. The sensitivity of the serological test for CD was 100%. In the four patients with CD, RSG improved liver function in two cases and stabilised liver function in one. The median follow-up was 16 months [16; 48 months]. Our work is interesting because it prospectively studies patients with proven cirrhosis and determines the prevalence of CD on the basis of CD serology and duodenal biopsy (Pr Azzouz has put a question mark over this - shall I delete it?). However, work on a larger scale and with longer follow-up is needed to study the maintenance of the improvement in liver function under RSG over time and the evolution of cirrhosis (regression, stabilisation, progression). Further studies are also needed to determine whether CD increases the risk of cirrhosis and to verify the accuracy of the 100% specificity of anti-EMA antibodies in screening for CD in cirrhotic patients. The fact that CD is present in cirrhotic patients with other aetiologies explaining the liver damage suggests a concomitant finding rather than a specific effect on the liver, but this remains to be demonstrated. The association between cryptogenic cirrhosis and CD also remains to be demonstrated by screening studies for CD in patients with cirrhosis of undetermined aetiology. In what follows, we propose to review the pathophysiology of CD and liver damage in CD. We will then review the literature on the association between CD and various chronic liver diseases.

## A- Reminder

### 1) Definition of celiac disease :

CD is defined by the European Society of Paediatrics, Gastroenterology, Hepatology and Nutrition as an autoimmune enteropathy secondary to the ingestion of gluten, a protein derived from wheat, rye and barley in genetically predisposed individuals (HLA-DQ2 or DQ8)[7] . It is characterised by chronic inflammation of the small intestine leading to villous atrophy, which impairs intestinal digestion and absorption. Diagnosis of CD in adults is based on celiac serology and intestinal histology.

RSG is currently the only treatment available. This purely dietary treatment leads to a regression of symptoms, an improvement in nutritional status and healing of the intestinal mucosa. Symptoms may be digestive or extra-digestive, or even absent; the latter two situations are currently the most common, making diagnosis more difficult [6].

**2) Prevalence of coeliac disease:**

It is a common disease, with a reported prevalence of around 1 in 200 to 1 in 100 in Europe and the United States, and 1 in 300 in Ireland. In North Africa, it is close to that observed in Europe, particularly in Tunisia, where it is estimated at 1/700 in blood donors (screened by auto-Ac)[8] (fig 3). In cirrhotic patients, the prevalence of CD is at least twice as high as in the general population[9, 10]. In our study, the prevalence of CD among cirrhotics is estimated at 1%, i.e. 7 times the prevalence of CD in the general Tunisian population. There are two peaks in the incidence of CD, the first in childhood, the second in adults between the ages of 20 and 40. However, the diagnosis may be made later, with 20% of adult forms diagnosed after the age of 60. CD predominantly affects women, with a sex ratio of 2 to 3:1, for which there is no clear explanation.In our study, all our CD patients were male and ranged in age from 20 to 48 years.

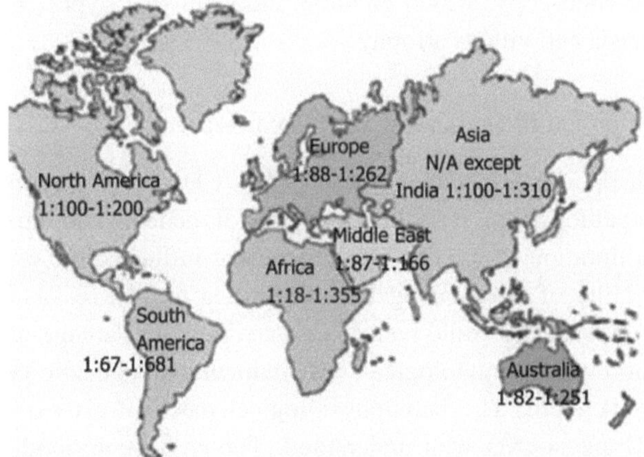


**Figure 3**: Prevalence of CD worldwide, NA: not available, Adapted from Gujral et al [11, 12].

## 3) Pathophysiology of celiac disease :

CD is the result of the interaction between gluten, favourable environmental factors and genetic predisposition. The initiator is gliadin, an antigen derived from the digestion of gluten by enzymes in the intestinal lumen and the brush border of enterocytes. Gliadin is responsible for activating innate immunity in the epithelium and adaptive immunity in the lamina propria. In the intestinal epithelium, gliadin causes lesions in the enterocytes, resulting in increased production of interleukin (IL)-15, which activates intraepithelial lymphocytes. Furthermore, during infection (e.g. by rotavirus) or in the presence of other factors that increase intestinal permeability, gliadin crosses the intestinal epithelial barrier and penetrates the lamina propria, where it is deaminated by tissue transglutaminase (TGt) and interacts with proteins of the HLA system on the surface of antigen-presenting cells. In individuals with the HLA-DQ2/DQ8 genotype, the presentation of gliadin in this HLA environment by APCs to specific CD4+ T lymphocytes leads to the production of pro-inflammatory cytokines, in particular gamma interferon, and the activation of B lymphocytes, producing antibodies against gliadin, but also against autoantigens (TTG and EMA).Taken together, these immunological phenomena lead to the histological abnormalities characteristic of CD observed in duodenal biopsies taken during upper digestive endoscopy, which combine intraepithelial hyperlymphocytosis, cryptic hyperplasia and villous atrophy.

## 4. Pathophysiology of liver damage in celiac disease:

The different hepatic manifestations observed in CD are most probably due to the same aetiopathogenies. It is the interplay of genetic and immunological factors and the duration of exposure to gluten that influence the effect of GFD and the reversibility of liver damage. It would therefore be reasonable to think that early diagnosis of CD could result in reversible liver damage under GVHD before interaction with immunological, environmental and genetic factors render the damage irreversible. The pathophysiological mechanisms explaining liver damage in CD are not yet well understood. The pathogenic models proposed are based on hypotheses rather than experimental studies [13]. The mechanism of liver damage is thought to be multifactorial, involving :

1) Malabsorption and chronic malnutrition
2) Increased intestinal permeability
3) The role of intestinal bacterial flora

4) Intestinal inflammation
5) Genetic predisposition

**4a Malabsorption and chronic malnutrition :**

Damage to the integrity of the intestinal mucosa during CD is at the origin of the malabsorption syndrome which, if severe, leads to malnutrition. Although malnutrition is currently rarely observed in CD, it may interfere with the development of liver lesions, principally steatosis, in gluten-sensitive enteropathies[14].

**4b. Increased intestinal permeability** :

Liver damage in CD may be due to increased intestinal permeability. The oral lactulose/mannitol absorption test was significantly higher in CD patients with disturbed liver function than in those with normal liver function[13]. It is linked on the one hand to intestinal inflammation and on the other to increased secretion of zonulin, a molecule that regulates cell junctions of the "On the one hand, this leads to the formation of a 'tight-junction', and on the other, to the penetration of toxins, antigens and inflammatory substances (cytokines) into the portal circulation and exposure of the liver to these potentially hepatotoxic substances (Figure 4). However, liver dysfunction is also seen in patients with chronic inflammatory bowel disease, cow's milk enteropathy and food allergy, suggesting that it is not gluten that is the cause, but rather damage to the mucosa that leads to liver dysfunction [94]. Contrary to this hypothesis, patients with tropical sprue who have similar intestinal damage, including increased intestinal permeability, do not present liver enzyme abnormalities as often as the patien carriers with CD[15]

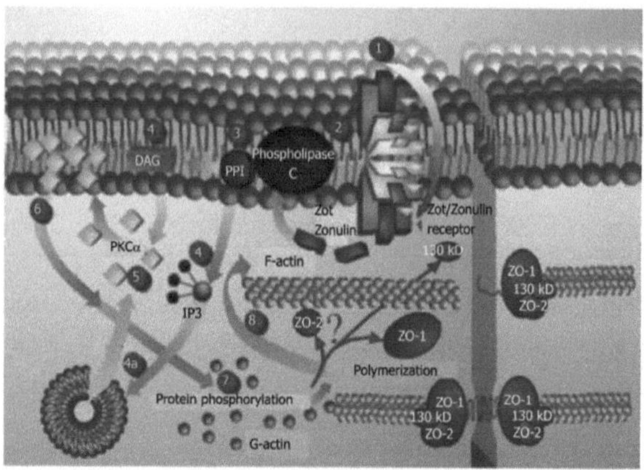


**Figure 4: Mechanism of the increase in intestinal permeability** (after Gujral et al[12, 16])1: Zot interacts with the intestinal Zot/Zonulin receptor. 2: protein internalisation; 3: activation of phospholipase C; 4: hydrolysis of phosphatidyl inositol to inositol 1,4,5-tris phosphate (PPI-3) and diacylglycerol (DAG); 5: activation of protein kinase C alpha (PKCa); 6: activated PKCa catalyses phosphorylation of target proteins; 7: sequential polymerisation of soluble G-actin into actin filaments; 8: this polymerisation leads to the rearrangement of tight junction (TJ) filaments and the displacement of proteins [including zonula occludens-1 (ZO-1)].As a result, Tight Junctions (TJs) become loose. IP3: Inositol trisphosphate.


## 4c. Role of the intestinal bacterial flora :

The growth of intestinal bacterial flora has been reported to be an aetiological factor that may be involved in liver dysfunction secondary to CD. In fact, the increase in intestinal transit time during untreated CD is at the origin of the growth of the bacterial flora and therefore of an increase in the intestinal antigen pool, which will be reabsorbed and discharged into the portal blood[5]. Kupffer cells play a pivotal role in the regulation of the immune response to bacterial antigens of intestinal origin[17].

## 4d.intestinal inflammation :

Chronic inflammation of the intestinal mucosa in CD leads to exposure of the TTG antigen (the main antigen in CD). TTG is ubiquitous throughout the body, including liver tissue. Recently, it has been shown that TTG type A antibodies can reach Ag TG in extra-intestinal tissues[18]. Their presence was shown in liver biopsies from two CD patients with hypertransaminasemia, thus consolidating the hypothesis that these antibodies could have a pathogenic role in the occurrence of extra-intestinal manifestations during CD and particularly liver damage, but this has never been demonstrated[18].

It is currently accepted that the risk of developing autoimmune diseases in CD increases with the duration of exposure to gluten and that the early introduction of GFDs protects against the development of immune disorders in CD, including liver dysfunction[19]. Thus, Prolonged exposure to gluten, secondary to late diagnosis, may explain the evolution of liver lesions, ranging from cryptogenic damage reversible under GFD to autoimmune hepatopathy which does not respond to GFD.

## 4e. Genetic predisposition :

Genetic predisposition plays an important role in favouring the progression of liver damage from cryptogenic lesions to irreversible autoimmune liver damage. It is currently well known that there is a common genetic predisposition between CD and certain dysimmune hepatopathies. In fact, the main genetic marker for CD is the HLA-DQ2 molecule, which is present in approximately 95% of patients with CD, the remainder being HLA-DQ8 positive[20]. From a genetic point of view, there is a strong link between the HLA DQ2 molecule and the HLA DR3 molecule, the latter being the main risk factor for the development of autoimmune hepatitis. Furthermore, in patients with PSC associated with chronic inflammatory bowel disease, the HLA-B8/DR3 molecule is frequently present. Thus, there is an HLA-type genetic correlation between CD, HAI and PSC; this has not been demonstrated with PBC[21]. Figure 5 summarises the pathophysiological mechanisms of liver damage in coeliac disease.

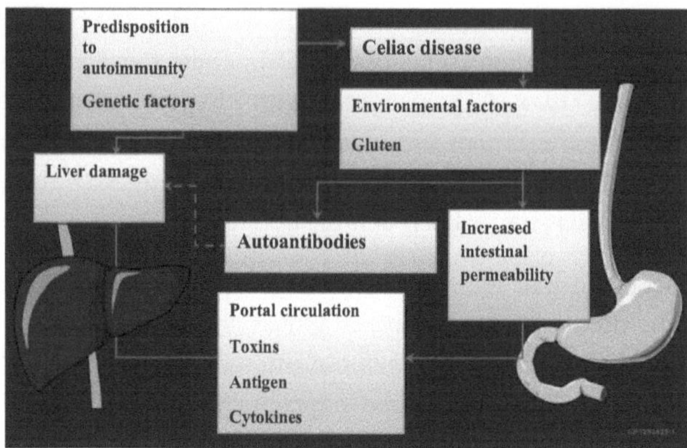



**Figure 5:** Pathophysiological mechanisms of liver damage in coeliac disease (after Rubio-Tapia et al[22]).

**B. Association between celiac disease and primary sclerosing cholangitis**

The relationship between CD and PSC is less well established. The first case reported in the literature dates from 1988, by Hay et al[23], who described three cases of patients with PSC (confirmed by endoscopic retrograde cholangiopancreatography and PBH) with steatorrhea and severe malabsorption, in whom the diagnosis of CD had been made secondarily. The diarrhoea regressed on RSG but the PSC did not improve. Since then, several cases have been reported in the literature (table12).

**Table 12**: Reported cases of the association of coeliac disease and primary sclerosing cholangitis

| Type of study | from | Number of patients | Symptoms | AC | Duodenal biopsy | Reply to the RSG | PBH | ERCP | Comorbidities | | Country/year | Reference |
|---|---|---|---|---|---|---|---|---|---|---|---|---|
| Reported cases | | 3 | Weight loss Steatorrhea | No | Typical | Yes | Yes | Yes | 2 RCH | | United States - United States 1988[23] | Hay et al |
| Case reported | | 69 | | 55% AGA+ | 0/26 Pathological | - | - | - | - | | Ireland 1992[19] | MacMatna et al |
| Reported cases | | 1 | Weight loss Diarrhoea Delayed of growth | No | Typical | Yes | Yes | Yes | Colitis chronic, Turner syndrome | from | France 1995[24] | Lacaille et al |
| Case reported | | 2 | Anemia | IgA AGA+ | Atrophy villous | Yes | Yes | Yes | - | | Italy 1996[25] | Fracassetti et al |
| Case reported | | 1 | Diarrhoea | No | Atrophy villous | Yes | Yes | Yes | RCH | | Sweden 1994[15] | Tysk et al |
| Case reported | | 1 | Folate deficiency | AG A- EM A+ | Atrophy villous | Yes | Yes | Yes | RCH Thyroiditis | | France 1994[17] | Brazier et al |
| Case reported | | 2 | Weight loss | EM A+ | Typical | Yes | Yes | Yes | - | | Italy 1998[26] | Venturini et al[ |
| Reported cases | | 1 | Anemia | No | NM | NM | yes | Yes | BY | | United States - United States 2001[27] | Gowet al[ |

| | | | | | | | | | | |
|---|---|---|---|---|---|---|---|---|---|---|
| Reported cases | 1 | Diarrhoea | TTG+ EMA- | Atrophy | NM | yes | NM | NM | Finland 2002[28] | Kaukinen Protruding EmA et al |
| Case reported | 2 | Screening from MC | EMA+ TTG+ | Typical | Yes | Yes | Yes | RCH | Poland 2002[29] | Habior et al [ |
| Prospective cohort | 69 | Screening from MC | 1,6% EMA 3.3% TTG | 100% Typical | Yes | Yes | Yes | - | Italy/ Spain 2002[30] | Volta et al |
| Reported cases | 2 | Weight loss Steatorrhea | EMA+ | Atrophy | Yes | No | Yes | RCH | United States - United States 2003[31] | Wurm et al |
| Case | 1 | Fortuitous | AGA+ | Typical | Yes | Yes | Yes | - | United States - | Al-Osaimi |
| reported | | | EMA+ | | | | | | Unis2 00 4 [32] | et al |
| Case reported | 1 | Diarrhoea | EMA+ | Typical | Yes | Yes | Yes | - | Spain 2005[33] | Cadahía et al |
| Prospective cohort | 155 | Screening | 3% EMA 9% TTG | - | - | - | - | - | United States 200 8 [10] | Rubio-Tapia et al |
| Case reported | 1 | Anemia Statural delay | TTG+ | Typical | Yes | Yes | No | No/MRI | Arabia Saudi 2013[34] | Al-Hussaini et al |

Typical: atrophy, crypt hyperplasia, intraepithelial lymphocytosis, AGA: anti-gliadin antibodies, ERCP: endoscopic retrograde cholangiopancreatography, RAP: rheumatoid arthritis, NM: not mentioned. On the basis of the data in the literature reporting fewer than 20 cases of PSC and CD, it is not legitimate to establish a genuine association between the two diseases. This association could be investigated by testing for CD (CD serology and duodenal biopsy) in patients with PSC and performing cholangiography in patients with CD[35].

MacMathuna et al [19] conducted a study of 69 patients with PSC and found that 55% of patients had positive anti-gliadin antibodies but intestinal biopsies did not show typical abnormalities in all patients. Rubio-Tapia et al [10] evaluated 155 patients with advanced PSC; those who expressed HLA-DQ2 or HLA-DQ8 had a high prevalence of CD antibodies: 9% of them were anti-TTG positive and 3% were anti-Ema positive. In view of these studies, the diagnosis of CD in patients with PSC requires awareness of the possible coexistence of the two diseases[35]. At present, screening f o r  CD using serology in patients with PSC cannot be routinely recommended [15, 17, 19, 23, 24, 34].


**C. Association between coeliac disease and primary biliary cholangitis:**

The first case of association of CD with PBC was published by Logan et al in 1978[36]. Four patients presented with symptoms suggestive of CD with a typical histological appearance on jejunal biopsy and improvement on GAS. Subsequently, an association between these two diseases has been widely reported in the literature and investigated in screening studies[37, 38].

In an English epidemiological study published in 1998 involving 250,000 individuals over a period of 12 years, a register of patients with PBC and those with CD showed that CD was present in 6 per cent of patients. % (4 out of 67) of patients with PBC [39].Conversely, in the same study, 3% (4 out of 143) of patients with CD had PBC. In an Irish study, Dickey et al [40] reported that the incidence of CD in PBC was at least 10 times that in the general population. Sorensen et al [41] reported an incidence rate of 27.6 in Denmark and 25.1 in Sweden. Contradictory results have been published in Sweden[42] , Italy[43, 44] and Greece[45] , which have not shown an increased risk of CD in patients with PBC. According to Bizzaro et al[46], 26% of patients with PBC are positive for anti-TTG Ac (ELISA assay). However, a true association was present in only 22% of cases in which anti-endomysial Ac was positive and the histology was typical of CD. Furthermore, Floreni et al[47] reported a high frequency of false positive anti-TTG antibodies in patients with PBC: 27.5%. of PBCs had anti-TTG AC levels above the upper limit of normal, of these, only two patients had anti-TTG levels >30 IU and anti-EMA Ac positivity was detected in only 3.4% of patients. Both authors therefore suggest that the false positivity of anti-TTG antibodies was due to the type of substrate used for the TTG assay. In fact, a high titre of anti-TTG antibodies is specific to CD, whereas lower titres may be seen in other gastrointestinal and liver diseases, and they therefore suggest that anti-EMA antibodies should always be added to the assay in PBC patients with positive anti-TTG antibodies. Studies of CD screening are listed in Table n°14.In countries where the prevalence of CD is low, the value of screening for CD in the absence of clinical suspicion in patients with PBC is questionable. Furthermore, RSG has not been shown to improve liver function in patients with coexisting PBC[36, 48]. Neuberger[49] reported the cases of two patients with PBC who were referred to a liver transplant centre (TH) in the United States because of deterioration in their liver function. These patients were asthenic and had chronic diarrhoea, and were diagnosed with CD and started on RSG. Progression was marked by improvement in liver function and TH was no longer necessary. Abnevolt et al [50] reported the case of a patient with CD, PBC and Helicobacter pylori infection, in whom a short period of GFD combined with ursodeoxycholic acid (AUDC) and anti-HP therapy resulted in marked improvement in the immunological status and histological lesions of PBC. In addition, Sedlack et al[51] showed clinical and biochemical improvement with RSG and AUDC. However, it is important to mention that the patient was taking the recommended treatment for PBC and that this improvement could be due to AUDC and not RSG.Several theories have been put forward to explain the concomitant presence of the two diseases: CD and PBC. It has been proposed that PBC is favoured by increased intestinal permeability[52, 53] and the same predisposition to autoimmunity. Screening for CD in patients with PBC is currently recommended because GFD can improve digestive symptoms and reduce the risk of cancer, osteoporosis and other autoimmune diseases[54, 55].

**Table13:** Reported cases of the association of coeliac disease and primary biliary cholangitis

| Association between PBC and CD: cases reported in the literature | | | | | | | | | |
| --- | --- | --- | --- | --- | --- | --- | --- | --- | --- |
| Number of patients | symptoms | Serology MC | Duodenal biopsy | RSG response | PBH | AMA | Comorbidities | Country /year | Reference |
| 4 | Weight loss Anemia, Diarrhoea | No | Typical | Yes | Yes | + | IgA deficiency | Scotland 1978 | Logan al[36] and |
| 1 | Weight loss Diarrhoea | No | Typical | Yes | Yes | No | - | United States 1978 | Lee et al[37] |
| 1 | Malabsorption | No | Typical | Mal compliance | Yes | + | - | Canada 1979 | Iliffe et al[56] |
| 1 | Diarrhoea Anemia | - | Atrophy subtotal | Yes | Yes | + | - | Ireland 1983 | Shanahan et al[48] |
| 1 | Dermatitis herpetiform | No | Typical | Yes | Yes | + | Dermatitis herpetiform | Norway 1985 | Gabriel sen al[57] and |
| 1 | Anemia | AGA- | Typical | Yes | Yes | + | Acidosis tubular | Ireland 1987 | Whitehead al[58] and |
| 1 | Weight loss Diarrhoea | No | Typical | Yes | Yes | + | - | United States 1992[59] | |
| 1 | Weight loss Anemia | No | Typical | Yes | Yes | + | - | Canada 1994 | Freeman[60] |
| 1 | Diarrhoea | No | Typical | Yes | Yes | + | - | Germany 1994 | Lohr et al[61] |
| 1 | Diarrhoea, Weight loss | AGA+ | Typical | No | Yes | + | - | Spain 1994 | Galvez al[61] and |
| 1 | Weight loss Steatorrhea | AGA+, EMA+ | Typical | Yes | Yes | + | Pullulation microbial | United States 1998 | Diabaise al[38] and |
| 1 | Anemia | EMA+ | Typical | Yes | Yes | No | - | United States 2002 | Sedlack al[51] and |
| 1 | Diarrhoea Weight loss | EMA+ | Typical | Yes | Yes | + | Renal tubular acidosis of gougerotsj ögren | Italy 2004 | Fracchia al[62] and |
| 1 | Anemia | AGA- EMA- | Typical | Yes | Yes | + | Osteomalacia, Myopathy | Turkey 2008 | Demirag al[63] and |
| 1 | Bone pain | AGA+ EMA+ | Typical | Yes | Yes | + | Fanconi syndrome Fanconi | France 2008 | Terrier et al[64] |

| 1 | | TTG+ | | | | | | | |
|---|---|---|---|---|---|---|---|---|---|
| 1 | Dyspepsia | TTG+ | Typical | Yes | Yes | + | Helicobacter pylori | Italy 2010 | Abnevoli and al[50] |
| 1 | Diarrhoea, Abdominal bloating | EMA + TTG+ | Typical | Yes | Yes | + | | India 2013 | Lodh et al[65] |

**Table14:** Screening studies for celiac disease in patients with primary biliary cholangitis

| Study | Screening method | Number of positive cases | Duodenal biopsy typical | Responseto the RSG | Country/year | Reference |
|---|---|---|---|---|---|---|
| Foresight | Duodenal biopsy | 5/6(19,2%) | 19,2% | No improvement inbalance sheet liver | Sweden 1982 | Olsson and al[66] |
| Retrospective | Diagnosis of PBC precedes CD | 2/18(11,1%) | Not mentioned | No improvement, either biological or histological | Sweden 1985 | Lofgren and al[67] |
| Foresight | EMA IF>1.5 | 6/57(11%) EMA | 7% | No improvement inbalance sheet liver | Ireland 1997 | Dickey and al[67] |
| Prospective cohort | AGA IgG, IgA>1AU IgA EMA IFI | 0/62 (0%) EMA+ 11/62(16%) AGA+ | 0/0 | - | United States, Italy | Volta and al[43] |
| Foresight | Malabsorption, AGA+ or family history of CD | 4/67(6%) | 4/67(6%) | No improvement inbalance sheet liver | United States 1998 | Kingham and al[39] |
| Foresight | AGA: IgA> 25 IU/mL, IgG> 28 IU/mL EmA IFI > 1:5 | 4/11 (36,4%) AGA IgA (+), 1/11 (9%) AGA IgG (+) 1/11 (9%) EmA (+) | 18% | - | Argentina 1998 | Niveloni al [68] and |
| Retrospective | EMA IFI > 1:5, TTGIgA ELISA > 140 IU/mL | 10/378 (2.6%) EMA (+) TTG (+), 44/378(11.6%) EMA (-) + TTG (+) | 1.30% | - | United States 2000 | Gillett and al[69] |

| Foresight | EMA IFI IgA TTG > 10 IU | 3/87 (3.4%) EMA (+) 24/87 (27.5%) TTG (+) | 0/17 | - | Italy, 2002 | Floreani and al[69] |
| Foresight | AGA IgA > 50 IU/mL, AGA IgG > 50 IU/ML EMA IgA IFI ≥ 1:5 IgA TTG> 30 IU/mL | 13/62 (21%) AGA (+) 0/62 EMA (+) 6/62 (10%) TTG (+) | 0/10 | - | Greece 2002 | Chatzicostas et al[45] |
| CohortProspective | IgA TTG > 7 IU/ml AGA IFI | 7/173 (4%) EmA (+) 5/173 (2.9%) TTG (+) | 7/7 | No improvement inbalance sheet liver | Italy/Spain 2002 | Volta et al[30] |
| CohortProspective | IgA anti-TTG> 7 UI IgG anti-TTG> 30 UI EMA IFI AGA Elisa | 7/115 (6.1%) TTG (+) 1/115 (0.9%) EMA (+) 8/115 (7.0%) AGA (+) | 1/8 | Improvement in duodenal histology | Poland, 2003 | Habior et al[70] |
| Prospective cohort | TTG ELISA | 28/105 (26.7%) IgA TTG(+) 6/105 (5.7%) IgG TTG(+) | 100%EmA(+) 0% TTG (+) | - | Italy, 2006 | Bizarro et al[46] |

**D. Association between celiac disease and autoimmune hepatitis:** The first cases of an association between CD and HAI were described in the late 1970s and early 1980s, followed by larger studies. The diagnosis of HAI in the initial studies was based on the presence of antibodies, typical histological lesions and hypergammaglobulinaemia in the absence of viral markers. Since the 1990s, a diagnostic score for HAI has been established[71].CD and HAI are associated with specific HLA class II genotypes: HLA DQ2/DQ8 for CD, HLA-DR3/DR4/DR52 for HAI [7]. These alleles may be found in combination (haplotypes) with varying frequency. The HLA-B8DR3 region in particular shows an imbalance of linkage with HLA-DQ2 and these two alleles are combined in a haplotype which is common in the Caucasian population. The preferential association of these alleles within these haplotypes could explain the shared genetic predisposition between CD and HAI[72]. An important feature is that actin-type anti-smooth muscle CAs are present in 90% of children and 60% of adults with CD [73, 74].Thus, in the presence of CD with altered liver enzymes, the positivity of anti-actin Ac may reflect villous atrophy and not be diagnostic of HAI[75]. The coexistence of two pathologies has been declared in the EASL consensus[76].

The incidence of HAI in adults with CD is 1.6% and in children 2% [77, 78], while the prevalence of CD in patients with HAI is ten times that of the general population [79]. The effect of RSG on liver function in patients with HAI is uncertain[5, 80]. However, a long-term beneficial effect of GFD is likely given that patients with HAI and CD have fewer relapses when immunosuppressive drugs are stopped compared with patients with HAI unrelated to CD[81, 82]. Screening for CD in patients with HAI is currently strongly recommended[83, 84]. Table 15 summarises published studies on the association of CD and HAI.

**Table 15:** Case reports on the association between coeliac disease and autoimmune hepatitis

| Cases reported in the literature on the association between HAI and CD | | | | | | | | |
|---|---|---|---|---|---|---|---|---|
| Number of patients | Symptoms | AC (HAI) | AC (MC) | Duodenal biopsy | Response to the RSG | Liver biopsy | Comorbidity | Country/ Author/ year |
| 1 | Anemia Infection | AMM :1/500 Anti-vimentine :1/500 | AGA IgG and IgA+ EMA + | Typical | Yes₂ | Chronic hepatitis active | Erythrobl-astopenia | France 2001 Bridoux Henno et al [85] |
| 1 | Weight loss Asthenia, Abdominal pain, Diarrhoea | ANA=1/1280 PANCA :1/2560 SMA :1/1200 LKM1 :1/50 | Ac anti reticulin 1/2000 , IgG+ AGA | Typical | No : developed HAI despite RSG | Chronic inflammation of portal region + ductular ductular + nodule of regeneration | Thyrotoxico se | Finland2002 Arvola et al[86] |
| 2 | Diarrhoea, Abdominal distension | ANA+, SMA+, anti-actin+ | ? | ? | Case 1: poor response to RSG Case 2 : developed HAI despite RSG | Hepatitis acute, pond necrosis, peri-portal lymphocytic infiltrate | - | Italy 2003 Leonard et al[87] |

| 1 | Cytolysis, Purpura, Hypoaesthesia of the t he le ft leg Skin ulcer two legs | ANA+ | AGA+ EMA + | Typical ₁ | Poor adhesionto RSG | Chronic active hepatitis mo derate, lesion inte rface hepatitis+po rtal fibrosis+prol iferation ductular | Cryoglo bulinemi a | Switz erlan d 2003 Bieck er et al[88 ] |
| 1 | Jaundice, d iscoloured stools | Negative, probable score | AGA IgA+ AGAI gG + EMA+ TTG IgA+ | Typical ₁ | Progressio n of liver damage despite the RSG | Moderate to severe lobular inflammatio n + hepatitis interface+fib rosis portale | - | Italy 2004 Iorio and al [89] |
| 1 | Anemia, Cytolysis | Negative | TTG+ | Villi atrophy | Elevation tr ansaminas es despite RSG | Severe lymphocytic inflammator y infiltration, patchy necrosis | - | Peru 2006 Tagle et al and [90] |
| 1 | Anorexia, Severe diarrhoea, Rapid weight loss | ANA+ SMA+ | EMA+ | Typical ₁ | A developed A cirrhosis despite GMS | Cirrhosis | Holmes-Adie syndrom e | Hung ary 2006 Csak et al[91 ] |
| 1 | Amenorrh oea, Anaemia, Jaundice | SMA+ | TTG IgA and IgG+, AGA+ , EMA+ . | Typical ₁ | Poor adhesion to the RSG | Confirms the diagnosis of HAI | Multiple sclerosis | Italy 2008 Ferro et al[92 ] |
| 1 | Weight loss Anorexia Asthenia Diarrhoea | ANA+++ | AGA (IgA IgG )+ EMA + TTG+ | Typical ₁ | Occurred of liver damage under RSG | Moderate chronic active hepatitis, interface hepatitis, portal fibrosis, ductopenia | Autoim mune thyroidit is Autoim mune cholangi tis | Turk ey 2009 Osasl an et al[93 ] |

| | | | | | | | | |
|---|---|---|---|---|---|---|---|---|
| 1 | malaise Intermittent vomiting rash osteopenia cytolysis | ANA,SMA LKM1 Anti mitochondria Anti LC1 ,Anti SLA/LP Anti parietal cells: are negative | TTG + | Typical[1] | Develops HAI under RSG | Lymphocytic hepatitis with moderate to severe activity | No | United States 2009 Quail et al [94] |
| 1 | 2abortions Joint pain Anaemia Asthenia Cytolysis | ANA+ì SMA+ AntiDNA: 0.1527778 | EMA :1/1 60 | Severe villous atrophy | Yes[2] | Active hepatitis with patchy necrosis an infiltrate periportal lymphocytic | Lupus | Italy 2010 Tovoli et al[95] |
| 1 | Anemia Asthenia Cytolysis liver | ANA :1/640 SMA :1/320 PANCA :1/160 | TTG+ ema+ | Villi atrophy | No, develops acute liver failure under RSG | Severe fibrosis | No | Italy 2013 Volta and al[96] |
| 1 | Unbalanced diabetes, Liver disorders | ANA :1/160 | Ig TTG+ EMA - | Typical[1] | Yes[2] | Chronic inflammation, interface hepatitis, patchy necrosis | Autoimmune thyroiditis diabetes[1] | Spain 2016 Dieli-crimi et al[97] |

1: villous atrophy + crypt hyperplasia + lymphoplasmacytic infiltrate; 2: patient treated with corticosteroids + azathioprine. AGA: Anti-gliadin antibody, SMA: Anti-smooth muscle antibody

**E. Association between coeliac disease and chronic hypertransaminasemia:**
Elevation of transaminases in addition to other causes of liver disease such as NASH, viral hepatitis, HAI, ethyl hepatitis and other rare genetic and metabolic causes is a frequent clinical situation[98].

Studies suggest that 10% of cryptogenic chronic hepatitis is due to CD [99, 100]. O n  the other hand, hypertransaminasemia has been reported in 9 to 40% of patients with CD[101, 102]. Multiple studies have shown that serum transaminase levels normalise in 75% to 95% of patients after 6 to 12 months on this diet[102] (table 16).

**Table 16:** Prevalence of hypertransaminasemia in patients with celiac disease and effect of GFD on this hypertransaminasemia

| Studies on the prevalence of hypertransaminasemia in patients with celiac disease (CD) and the effect of the gluten-free diet (GFD). | | | |
|---|---|---|---|
| Reference | Number of patients | Hypertransaminasemia (n, (%)) | Response to RSG (%) |
| | 74 | 29(39) | 100 |
| Hagander et al, 1977[103] | | | |
| | 132 | 62(47) | 75 |
| Jacobsen et al, 1990 [104] | | | |
| | 158 | 67(42) | 90 |
| Bardella et al, 1995[105]. | | | |
| | 129 | 19(15) | 79 |
| Dickey et al, 1995 [106] | | | |
| | 178 | 72(40) | 89 |
| Novacek et al, 1999[77]. | | | |
| | 99 | 34(34) | 63 |
| Foley et al, 2009 [107] | | | |
| | 572 | 60(11) | Not reported |
| Lewis et al, 2009[108] | | | |
| | 313 | 33(11) | Not reported |
| Korpimakiet al, 2011[109]. | | | |
| | 65 | 37(57) | 95 |
| Bonamicoand al, 1986 (paediatric)[110]. | | | |
| | 114 | 37(32) | 100 |
| Farre et al, 2002 (paediatric)[111]. | | | |
| | 27 | 7(26) | 100 |
| Arslan et al, 2005 (paediatric)[112]. | | | |

Histological abnormalities in patients who had undergone an initial PBH were also regressive with RSG [104].

## F. Association between celiac disease and non-alcoholic steatohepatitis

NASH is a major cause of chronic liver disease, with a worldwide prevalence estimated at 24% [113].The high prevalence of obesity worldwide has influenced the economic burden of NASH[114]. In the absence of metabolic syndrome, NASH may be linked to the concomitant presence of CD. CD patients have a high risk of developing NASH compared with the general population[115]. Approximately 3% of CD patients with histologically proven

NASH show normalisation of liver enzymes after 6 months of GFR[116, 117]. Given the frequency of sub-clinical or silent presentations of CD, CD antibody testing should be performed in the presence of NASH and in the absence of metabolic risk factors and other causes of chronic liver disease[118, 119].

**G. Association between celiac disease and viral hepatitis C :**

The hepatitis C virus (HCV) could be involved in breaking down immune tolerance to self-antigens and thus triggering auto-reactivity.
HCV has been implicated in the triggering of autoimmune diseases and in the formation of autoantibodies[120].
The association between CD and viral hepatitis C is currently controversial and needs to be clarified. Although some authors have reported a higher incidence of CD among patients with HCV[121], this association cannot be attributed to the presence of HCV. confirmed in low-prevalence regions[122]. Nevertheless, particular attention should be paid to HCV patients treated with interferon (INF), as studies have reported cases of CD occurring under this treatment, requiring its discontinuation[120]. As in the case of CD, patients placed on INF may present with severe diarrhoea, refractory anaemia and hypoferritinaemia. Thus, evoking CD in the presence of these symptoms as a differential diagnosis and making the diagnosis in time will allow appropriate management of the underlying disease[123]. Considering the data in the literature, screening for CD should be carried out before treatment is started. If serology is positive, IFN-free treatment should be preferred. If this treatment is not available, GFR should be initiated with close monitoring during the treatment period[121, 124].It should be noted that the interference between CD and the new antiviral treatment is not yet well known, but it seems to be a safer alternative given its mechanism of action.

**H. Association between celiac disease and viral hepatitis B :**

Studies assessing the coexistence of CD and viral hepatitis B have shown that there is no obvious association between these two diseases. In studies of HBV carriers screening for CD, the positivity rate of anti-EMA and anti-TTG antibodies varies between 0-8% and 0-10% respectively. Only 10% have histologically compatible lesions[125, 126].
Several studies have reported reduced efficacy of the HBV vaccine in patients with CD; this was confirmed by a recent meta-analysis[127]. New antiviral B

immunisation strategies have been proposed to ensure complete protection. These strategies include a an increase in the dose and/or an additional injection with intra-muscular or preferably intra-dermal administration. In addition, a booster dose after 10 years is recommended[127].


## I. Association between coeliac disease and non-cirrhotic portal hypertension:

The association of CD and idiopathic non-cirrhotic intrahepatic hypertension (NCHIHN) has been reported in the literature[128, 129], including one case of gastrointestinal haemorrhage from ruptured oesophageal varices[130]. It has been suggested that in CD, repetitive antigenic stimulation of the portal vein and the resulting immune response leads to idiopathic portal hypertension[131]. In India, 10% of patients with HPIHNC have histologically proven CD[132]. The rate of survival without liver transplantation decreases in the case of associated CD[133]. Based on current literature, all patients with unexplained portal hypertension should be screened for CD [132, 134], although there is no evidence that GSR can change the course of the disease or improve survival.

**Association between celiac disease and cirrhosis:** (Rq DR safer: review the results of our study and the literature, then discuss) Our study showed that the prevalence of CD in cirrhosis was seven times higher than in the general population, and that the introduction of GFDs led to an improvement in liver function. We also found that CD was particularly prevalent in cryptogenic cirrhosis. A review of the literature showed that CD is twice as common in cirrhotic patients as in the general population[4]. An association between CD and cryptogenic cirrhosis has also been suggested in the literature [135-137]. The absence of typical hepatic histological lesions in CD indicates that this disease does not directly damage the liver [138].

Cases of patients with decompensated cirrhosis who improved after the introduction of RSG and were even taken off the liver transplant list have been reported in the literature [34, 138, 139]. These data suggest that all cirrhotic patients, particularly those with hypo albuminemia and ascites [4, 138], should be screened for CD because, regardless of the etiology of cirrhosis, GSR has a beneficial effect in advanced liver disease with associated CD.

In a Finnish study, CD was found in four patients with advanced liver disease who were listed for liver transplantation. One patient had congenital fibrosis of the liver, another had massive hepatic steatosis and the other two had cryptogenic cirrhosis[28].Their liver function had improved with GFR (table17). This prompted the authors to conduct a screening study for CD in patients with severe liver disease listed for liver transplantation. This study involved 185 patients and found that 8 (4.3%) of them had CD, which corresponds to 4 to 10 times the prevalence of CD in Finland. Only one patient was put on a GFD. This suggests that in some cases, treatment with a GFD can prevent the onset of CD. liver transplantation [28].

**Table17:** Changes in liver function before and after dieting Finnish study 2002 (after Kaukinen et al[28])

| | Patient 1 | | Patient 2 | | Patient3 | | Patient4 | |
|---|---|---|---|---|---|---|---|---|
| | Before RSG | After RSG | Before RSG | After RSG | Before RSG | After RSG | Before RSG | After RSG |
| General condition | bad | Improved | bad | improved | bad | Improved | bad | Improved |
| Jaundice | +++ | 0 | + | +/- | 0 | 0 | 0 | 0 |
| Ascites | +++ | 0 | +++ | 0 | +++ | 0 | +++ | 0 |
| INR(0.9-1.2) | 3 | 1,3 | 1,5-1,1 | 1 | 2,1-1,1 | 1,1 | 1,1 | 1,3 |
| Albumin, g /l (>40g/L) | 18 | 41 | 16 | 38 | 12 | 44 | 29 | 37 |
| Bilirubin, umol/l (<20umol/l) | >500 | 25 | 40 | 31 | 13 | 8 | 25 | 24 |
| Alkaline phosphatase U/L(<50U/L) | 940 | 735 | 188 | 96 | 358 | 117 | 622 | 835 |
| ALT,U/L(<50U/L) | 3390 | 91 | 57 | 25 | 122 | 18 | 41 | 33-50 |
| Liver histology | Acute hepatitis | Improved | Fibrosis + Ductular proliferation | Not done | Steatosis50 | Improved | Cirrhosis + lymphocytic infiltration -ary moderate | Micronodular cirrhosis hepatitis chronicle |
| HLA type | HLA DQ2 | | Not done | | HLADQ2 | | HLA DQ2 | |

In another retrospective cohort of liver transplant patients conducted in the United States in 2008 [10] (310 patients with end-stage dysimmune liver disease and 178 patients with end-stage non-dysimmune liver disease), the prevalence of anti- The prevalence of Ac TTG and Ac anti-EMA was significantly higher in HLA DQ2 or HLA DQ8 patients with dysimmune liver disease compared with those without (14.2% versus 5.4%, P=0.0001 and 4.3% versus 0.78%,P=0.01 respectively).The prevalence of Ac TTG and EMA was 5 times higher in the group with dysimmune liver disease (3% versus 0.6%).As the study was retrospective, duodenal biopsies were performed in only two patients. Thus, the definitive diagnosis of CD cannot be made in patients with positive CD serology. The CD Ac assay performed at 6-12 or 24 months after liver transplantation normalised in 94% to 100% of cases respectively without exclusion of gluten. This suggests that negative CD serology post liver transplantation does not exclude the diagnosis of CD, thus reinforcing the value of screening for CD pre liver transplantation in patients with advanced liver disease[10].The association of cirrhosis and CD has also been described in children [136].Demir et al reported the case of five children with CD and cryptogenic cirrhosis. In three cases, the diagnosis of CD and cirrhosis was concomitant and in the other 2 cases, the diagnosis of CD preceded that of cirrhosis. After 1 to 5 years of GFD, clinical improvement and normalisation of liver enzymes were noted in three cases, whereas the other two were not compliant with GFD and therefore there was no improvement in liver function[136].Al-Hussaini et al [34] reported the case of an 11-year-old girl with hepatocellular failure secondary to PSC. Treatment with a combination of ursodeoxycholic acid, RSG and corticosteroids improved liver function. Cases of CD with liver failure requiring TH have also been reported. Pavon et al[140] reported the case of a 14 year old girl with CD who developed severe liver dysfunction requiring TH after a long course of exposure to gluten. Casswall et al [141] reported six cases of girls aged between 13 and 36 months with CD who developed severe liver dysfunction after 1 to 24 months of gluten exposure. After orthotopic TH, patients treated with mycophenolic acid may experience diarrhoea. Indeed, this treatment may induce histological lesions similar to CD. It is therefore important to differentiate between these two entities in order to guide appropriate management[142]. Given these data, a prospective study was conducted in the United States in 2014[4]. It looked at screening for CD in cirrhotic patients regardless of the underlying aetiology. The study included 204 patients with proven cirrhosis. CD serology and duodenal biopsy were performed systematically; 2.5% of cirrhotic patients were carriers of CD. This corresponds to twice the prevalence of CD in the general population in America. The sensitivity and specificity of TTG antibodies for the detection of CD were 80% and 100% respectively, and for EMA antibodies was 100%. The five patients with CD were three men and two women. The aetiologies of cirrhosis were: HAI, CSP, NASH, cryptogenic and alcoholic. All patients were treated with GVHD, which improved liver function in four cases. (table18)

**Table18:**Changes in liver function before and after gluten-free diet, United States 2014 (after Pagadala et al[4])

| | | Patient1 | | Patient2 | | Patient3 | | Patient4 | | Patient5 | |
|---|---|---|---|---|---|---|---|---|---|---|---|
| Gender | | Male | | Female | | Female | | Male | | Male | |
| Age (years) | | 62 | | 67 | | 53 | | 21 | | 59 | |
| Etiology | | NASH | | Cryptogenic | | CSP | | HAI | | Alcoholic | |
| Damage kidney | | Yes | | No | | No | | No | | No | |
| | | Pré RSG | Pos RSG | Pré RSG | Post RSG | Pré RSG | Post RSG | Pré RSG | Post RSG | Pré RSG | Post RSG |
| EMA | | >1/160 | <1/10 | >1/160 | <1/10 | >1/160 | <1/10 | 1/80 | <1/10 | 1/40 | NF |
| IgG gliadin | | 44 | NF | 139 | 98 | 42 | 4 | 62 | 19 | 18 | NF |
| IgA gliadin | | 51 | NF | 194 | 73 | 53 | 6 | 52 | 10 | 83 | NF |
| TTG | | 124 | NF | 103 | 17 | 175 | 1 | 12 | 5 | 139 | NF |
| Stadium of Marsh | | 3 | 0 | 3 | 0 | 3 | 0 | 3 | NF | 3 | NF |
| BMI | | 35 | 34 | 38 | 37 | 23,3 | 24,7 | 27,4 | 29,8 | 30 | NF |
| Bilirubin | | 0,9 | 0,3 | 2,2 | 1,7 | 0,6 | 0,4 | 18,8 | 1,1 | 1,3 | NF |
| ASAT | | 35 | 24 | 53 | 42 | 25 | 24 | 1497 | 24 | 82 | NF |
| ALAT | | 40 | 11 | 32 | 26 | 20 | 14 | 799 | 44 | 41 | NF |
| TP | | 8 | 7 | 7,2 | 6,8 | 9,1 | 8,5 | 7,4 | 7,2 | 12,7 | NF |
| Albumin | | 4 | 4,1 | 2,8 | 2,5 | 4,9 | 4,6 | 3,5 | 4 | 2,6 | NF |
| PA | | 367 | 114 | 156 | 155 | 178 | 129 | 138 | 65 | 145 | NF |
| INR | | 1 | 1 | 1,3 | 1,2 | 1,1 | 1 | 1,7 | 1,1 | 1,2 | NF |
| Creatinine | | 0,9 | 1,4 | 0,8 | 0,8 | 0,67 | 0,62 | 0,73 | 0,83 | 0,6 | NF |
| MELD | | 6 | 10 | 12 | 10 | 7 | 6 | 23 | 8 | 10 | NF |
| Deaths | | no | | No | | no | | No | | After 1 month of liver biopsy | |

PT: prothrombin rate, AP: alkaline phosphatase, NF: not done

The data from our study and from the literature show that CD is particularly more frequent in cirrhotic patients than in the general population, and that the introduction of RSG can improve liver function and take patients off the liver transplant list.

# CONCLUSION AND RECOMMENDATIONS

Hepatic impairment in CD represents a broad spectrum, with a continuum ranging from moderate hepatic impairment to severe hepatic dysfunction. It presents in two clinical forms: cryptogenic hepatopathy and dysimmune hepatopathy. Epidemiological studies have shown that the prevalence of CD in cirrhotic patients is higher than in the general population. It has also been shown that CD may be the cause of chronic cryptogenic liver disease, which may improve after the introduction of GFR even at the stage of cirrhosis. We conducted a prospective bi-centric study of patients with cirrhosis of various aetiologies hospitalised in the gastroenterology departments of the Fattouma Bourguiba University Hospital in Monastir and the Mohamed Taher Maamouri University Hospital in Nabeul. The aim of our study was to detect CD in cirrhotic patients and to evaluate the evolution of liver function after the introduction of GFR in positive cases. We included 100 patients in our study. There were 55 men and 45 women, with a mean age of 57 years. At the time of inclusion, 91% of the patients had decompensated cirrhosis. The aetiologies of cirrhosis were viral hepatitis B in 23 cases, viral hepatitis C in 14 cases, cryptogenic cirrhosis in 39 cases and cirrhosis secondary to NASH in 8 cases. The prevalence of CD in this study sample was 1%, which corresponds to seven times the prevalence of CD in the general population of our country. The sensitivity of anti-EMA antibodies to detect CD in our study was 100%. In all four patients with CD, cirrhosis was cryptogenic. We followed this patient for two years in order to assess the effect of RSG on liver function. This patient was 42 years old. He was admitted for management of a poorly tolerated anaemic syndrome. Investigations revealed a concomitant diagnosis of CD and cirrhosis. The patient was put on RSG. Progress was good, with clinical, biological and histological improvement. We also reported three cases of patients with CD and cirrhosis from two gastroenterology departments. The first patient was 39 years old with no specific pathological history. He was admitted for investigation of a chronic transit disorder with alternating diarrhoea and constipation. Clinical, biological, morphological and histological investigations led to a diagnosis of CD and cryptogenic cirrhosis. The patient was put on a well-monitored GFR with partial improvement in liver function. The second patient was aged 20 and had a family history of jaundice of undetermined aetiology. He was admitted with severe acute hepatitis in the setting of chronic liver disease at the stage of cirrhosis of undetermined aetiology. Celiac serology and duodenal biopsies were consistent with a diagnosis of celiac disease. The patient did not follow the GFD and died after 7 months of follow-up in sepsis with decompensation of cirrhosis. The third patient was 48 years old. He was admitted with oedemato-ascitic decompensation inaugurating cryptogenic cirrhosis. His history included gluten intolerance, but the patient was not properly monitored. He was put on a GFD with poor compliance. After 9 months of follow-up, he presented with a second oedemato-ascitic decompensation. The notion of poorly monitored CD in this patient implies that if the GFD had been started early, it could have prevented the worsening of the liver damage.

**Recommendations:**

Based on our results and a review of the literature, screening for CD should be recommended in cases of :

-autoimmune liver disease
-primary biliary cholangitis
- hepatic steatosis in the absence of metabolic syndrome
- cryptogenic cirrhosis
-Non-cirrhotic intrahepatic portal hypertension (NICPTH)
- patients listed for liver transplantation
In the case of viral hepatitis C, it is important to look for CD, as it presents a relative contraindication to interferon. RSG improves the symptoms associated with CD and may prevent the onset of other immunological disorders and degeneration. However, the associated liver damage may improve, stabilise or worsen.

# REFERENCES

1. Vahedi, K., Y. Bouhnik, and C. Matuchansky, Adult celiac disease. 2001.
2. Hankey, G. and G. Holmes, Coeliac disease in the elderly. Gut, 1994. **35**(1): p. 65-67.
3. Spijkerman, M., et al, A wide variety of clinical features and concomitant disorders in celiac disease - A cohort study in the Netherlands. Dig Liver Dis, 2016. **48**(5): p. 499-505.
4. Pagadala, M.R., et al, Prevalence of celiac disease in cirrhosis and outcome of cirrhosis on a gluten free diet: a prospective study. Journal of hepatology, 2014. **61**(3): p. 558-563.
5. Rubio-Tapia, A. and J.A. Murray, The liver in celiac disease. Hepatology, 2007. **46**(5): p. 1650- 1658.
6. Rubio-Tapia, A., et al, ACG clinical guidelines: diagnosis and management of celiac disease.
The American journal of gastroenterology, 2013. **108**(5): p. 656-676.
7. Husby, S., et al, European Society for Pediatric Gastroenterology, Hepatology, and Nutrition Guidelines for the Diagnosis of Coeliac Disease. Journal of Pediatric Gastroenterology and Nutrition, 2012. **54**(1): p. 136-160.
8. Bdioui, F., et al, Prevalence of celiac disease in Tunisian blood donors. Gastroentérologie Clinique et Biologique, 2006. **30**(1): p. 33-36.
9. Narciso-Schiavon, J.L. and L.L. Schiavon, To screen or not to screen? Celiac antibodies in liver diseases. World J Gastroenterol, 2017. **23**(5): p. 776-791.
10. Rubio-Tapia, A., et al, Celiac disease autoantibodies in severe autoimmune liver disease and the effect of liver transplantation. Liver International, 2008. **28**(4): p. 467-476.
11. Gujral, N., H.J. Freeman, and A.B. Thomson, Celiac disease: prevalence, diagnosis, pathogenesis and treatment. World J Gastroenterol, 2012. **18**(42): p. 6036-59.
12. Gujral, N., H.J. Freeman, and A.B. Thomson, Celiac disease: prevalence, diagnosis, pathogenesis and treatment. World journal of gastroenterology: WJG, 2012. **18**(42): p. 6036.
13. Volta, U., Pathogenesis and clinical significance of liver injury in celiac disease. Clin Rev Allergy Immunol, 2009. **36**(1): p. 62-70.
14. Freeman, H.J., Reproductive changes associated with celiac disease. World Journal of Gastroenterology, 2010. **16**(46): p. 5810.
15. Tysk, C., Concurrent ulcerative colitis, celiac sprue, and primary sclerosing cholangitis. Journal of clinical gastroenterology, 1994. **18**(3): p. 241.

16. Fina, D., et al, Interleukin 21 contributes to the mucosal T helper cell type 1 response in coeliac disease. Gut, 2008. **57**(7): p. 887-892.

17. Brazier, F., et al, Primary sclerosing cholangitis and coeliac disease: beneficial effect of gluten-free diet on the liver. European journal of gastroenterology & hepatology, 1994. **6**(2): p. 183-186.

18. Korponay-Szabo, I.R., In vivo targeting of intestinal and extraintestinal transglutaminase 2 by coeliac autoantibodies. Gut, 2004. **53**(5): p. 641-648.

19. Macmathuna, P., et al, Is gluten enteropathy common in chronic liver disease. Gastroenterology, 1992. **102**: p. A845.

20. Sollid, L.M. and E. Thorsby, HLA susceptibility genes in celiac disease: Genetic mapping and role in pathogenesis. Gastroenterology, 1993. **105**(3): p. 910-922.

21. Juran, B.D. and K.N. Lazaridis, Genetics and genomics of primary biliary cirrhosis. Clin Liver Dis, 2008. **12**(2): p. 349-65; ix.

22. Rubio-Tapia, A. and J.A. Murray, The liver in celiac disease. Hepatology, 2007. **46**(5): p. 1650- 8.

23. Hay, J.E., et al, Primary sclerosing cholangitis and celiac disease. Ann Intern Med, 1988. **109**:p. 713-717.

24. Lacaille, F., et al, Celiac disease, inflammatory colitis, and primary sclerosing cholangitis in a girl with Turner's syndrome. Journal of pediatric gastroenterology and nutrition, 1995. **21**(4): p. 463-467.

25. Fracassetti, O., et al, Primary sclerosing cholangitis with celiac sprue: two cases. Journal of clinical gastroenterology, 1996. **22**(1): p. 71-72.

26. Venturini, I., et al, Adult celiac disease and primary sclerosing cholangitis: two case reports. Hepato-gastroenterology, 1998. **45**(24): p. 2344-2347.

27. Gow, P.J., K.A. Fleming, and R.W. Chapman, Primary sclerosing cholangitis associated with rheumatoid arthritis and HLA DR4: is the association a marker of patients with progressive liver disease? Journal of hepatology, 2001. **34**(4): p. 631-635.

28. Kaukinen, K., et al, Celiac disease in patients with severe liver disease: gluten-free diet may reverse hepatic failure. Gastroenterology, 2002. **122**(4): p. 881-888.

29. Habior, A., et al, Association of primary sclerosing cholangitis, ulcerative colitis and coeliac disease in female siblings. European journal of

gastroenterology & hepatology, 2002. **14**(7):p. 787-791.

30. Volta, U., et al, Celiac disease in autoimmune cholestatic liver disorders. The American journal of gastroenterology, 2002. **97**(10): p. 2609-2613.

31. Wurm, P., A.D. Dixon, and B.J. Rathbone, Ulcerative colitis, primary sclerosing cholangitis and coeliac disease: two cases and review of the literature. European journal of gastroenterology & hepatology, 2003. **15**(7): p. 815-817.

32. Al-Osaimi, A.M. and C.L. Berg, Association of primary sclerosing cholangitis and celiac disease: a case report and review of the literature. The American Journal of Gastroenterology, 2002. **97**(9): p. S85.

33. Cadahia, V., et al, Celiac disease (CD), ulcerative colitis (UC), and primary sclerosing cholangitis (PSC) in one patient: a family study. Revista espanola de enfermedades digestivas: organo oficial de la Sociedad Espanola de Patologia Digestiva, 2005. **97**(12): p. 907-913.

34. Al-Hussaini, A., A. Basheer, and A.J. Czaja, Liver failure unmasks celiac disease in a child. Ann Hepatol, 2013. **12**: p. 501-505.

35. Schrumpf, E., Association of primary sclerosing cholangitis and celiac disease: fact or fancy?
Hepatology, 1989. **10**(6): p. 1020-1021.

36. Logan, R., et al, Primary biliary cirrhosis and coeliac disease: an association? The Lancet, 1978. **311**(8058): p. 230-233.

37. Gálvez, C., V. Garrigues, and J. Ponce, Primary biliary cirrhosis and coeliac disease. European Journal of Gastroenterology & Hepatology, 1994. **6**(9): p. B77.

38. DiBaise, J.K. and F.F. Paustian, Steatorrhea and weight loss in a 72-year-old man: Primary biliary cirrhosis? celiac disease? bacterial overgrowth? what else? The American journal of gastroenterology, 1998. **93**(11): p. 2226-2230.

39. Kingham, J. and D. Parker, The association between primary biliary cirrhosis and coeliac disease: a study of relative prevalences. Gut, 1998. **42**(1): p. 120-122.

40. Dickey, W., S.A. McMillan, and M.E. Callender, High prevalence of celiac sprue among patients with primary biliary cirrhosis. Journal of clinical gastroenterology, 1997. **25**(1): p. 328-329.

41. Sørensen, H.T., et al, Risk of primary biliary liver cirrhosis in patients with coeliac disease: Danish and Swedish cohort data. Gut, 1999. **44**(5): p. 736-738.

42. Sjöberg, K., S. Lindgren, and S. Eriksson, Frequent Occurrence of Non-Specific Gliadin Antibodies in Chronic Liver Disease Endomysial but Not Gliadin Antibodies Predict Coeliac Disease in Patients with Chronic Liver Disease. Scandinavian journal of gastroenterology, 1997. **32**(11): p. 1162-1167.

43. Volta, U., et al, Frequency and significance of anti-gliadin and anti-endomysial antibodies in autoimmune hepatitis. Digestive diseases and sciences, 1998. **43**(10): p. 2190-2195.

44. Bardella, M.T., et al, Screening patients with celiac disease for primary biliary cirrhosis and vice versa. American Journal of Gastroenterology, 1997. **92**(9).

45. Chatzicostas, C., et al, Primary biliary cirrhosis and autoimmune cholangitis are not associated with coeliac disease in Crete. BMC gastroenterology, 2002. **2**(1): p. 5.

46. Bizzaro, N., et al, Low specificity of anti-tissue transglutaminase antibodies in patients with primary biliary cirrhosis. Journal of clinical laboratory analysis, 2006. **20**(5): p. 184-189.

47. Floreani, A., et al, Prevalence of coeliac disease in primary biliary cirrhosis and of antimitochondrial antibodies in adult coeliac disease patients in Italy. Digestive and Liver Disease, 2002. **34**(4): p. 258-261.

48. Shanahan, F., P. O'Regan, and J. Crowe, Primary biliary cirrhosis associated with coeliac disease. Irish medical journal, 1983. **76**(6): p. 282.

49. Neuberger, J., PBC and the gut: the villi atrophy, the plot thickens. Gut, 1999. **44**(5): p. 594- 595.

50. Abenavoli, L., et al, Celiac disease, primary biliary cirrhosis and helicobacter pylori infection: one link for three diseases. International journal of immunopathology and pharmacology, 2010. **23**(4): p. 1261-1265.

51. Sedlack, R.E., et al, Celiac disease-associated autoimmune cholangitis. The American journal of gastroenterology, 2002. **97**(12): p. 3196-3198.

52. Feld, J.J., J. Meddings, and E.J. Heathcote, Abnormal intestinal permeability in primary biliary cirrhosis. Digestive diseases and sciences, 2006. **51**(9): p. 1607-1613.

53. Di Leo, V., et al, Gastroduodenal and intestinal permeability in primary biliary cirrhosis. European journal of gastroenterology & hepatology, 2003. **15**(9): p. 967-973.

54. Antvorskov, J.C., et al, Dietary gluten and the development of type 1 diabetes. Diabetologia, 2014. **57**(9): p. 1770-1780.

55. Cosnes, J., et al, Incidence of autoimmune diseases in celiac disease: protective effect of the gluten-free diet. Clinical Gastroenterology and Hepatology, 2008. **6**(7): p. 753-758.

56. Iliffe, G.D. and D.A. Owen, An association between primary biliary cirrhosis and jejunal villous atrophy resembling celiac disease. Digestive diseases and sciences, 1979. **24**(10): p. 802-806.

57. Gabrielsen, T. and P. Hoel, Primary biliary cirrhosis associated with coeliac disease and dermatitis herpetiformis. Dermatology, 1985. **170**(1): p. 31-34.
58. Fouin-Fortunet, H., et al, Celiac disease associated with primary biliary cirrhosis.
Clinical and Biological Gastroenterology, 1985. **9**(8-9): p. 641-642.
59. Ginn, P. and R. Workman, Primary biliary cirrhosis and adult celiac disease. Western journal of medicine, 1992. **156**(5): p. 547.
60. Freeman, H.J., Celiac Disease Associated with Primary Biliary Cirrhosis in a Coast Salish Native. Canadian Journal of Gastroenterology and Hepatology, 1994. **8**(2): p. 105-107.
61. Löhr, M., et al, Primary biliary cirrhosis associated with coeliac disease. European journal of gastroenterology & hepatology, 1994. **6**(3): p. 263-268.
62. Fracchia, M., et al, Coeliac disease associated with Sjögren's syndrome, renal tubular acidosis, primary biliary cirrhosis and autoimmune hyperthyroidism. Digestive and liver disease, 2004. **36**(7): p. 489-491.
63. Demirag, M.D., et al, Osteomalacic myopathy associated with coexisting coeliac disease and primary biliary cirrhosis. Medical Principles and Practice, 2008. **17**(5): p. 425-428.
64. Terrier, B., et al, Osteomalacia revealing celiac disease and primary biliary cirrhosis-related Fanconi syndrome in a patient with systemic sclerosis. Clinical and experimental rheumatology, 2007. **26**(3): p. 467-470.
65. Lodh, M., A.A. Ahmed, and D. Pradhan, A case of coexistent primary biliary cirrhosis and celiac disease. Indian Journal of Allergy, Asthma and Immunology, 2013. **27**(2): p. 138.
66. Olsson, R., I. Kagevi, and L. Rydberg, On the concurrence of primary biliary cirrhosis and intestinal villous atrophy. Scandinavian journal of gastroenterology, 1982. **17**(5): p. 625-628.
67. Loufgren, J., et al, Incidence and Prevalence of Primary Biliary Cirrhosis in a Denned Population in Sweden. Scandinavian journal of gastroenterology, 1985. **20**(5): p. 647-650.
68. Niveloni, S., et al, Gluten sensitivity in patients with primary biliary cirrhosis. The American journal of gastroenterology, 1998. **93**(3): p. 404-408.
69. Gillett, H.R., et al, Prevalence of IgA antibodies to endomysium and tissue transglutaminase in primary biliary cirrhosis. Canadian Journal of Gastroenterology and Hepatology, 2000. **14**(8): p. 672-675.
70. Habior, A., et al, Association of coeliac disease with primary biliary cirrhosis in Poland.
European journal of gastroenterology & hepatology, 2003. **15**(2): p. 159-164.

71. Johnson, P.J. and I.G. McFarlane, Meeting report: international autoimmune hepatitis group.
Hepatology, 1993. **18**(4): p. 998-1005.
72. Panetta, F., et al, Celiac Disease in Pediatric Patients with Autoimmune Hepatitis. Pediatric Drugs, 2012. **14**(1): p. 35-41.
73. Granito, A., et al, Antibodies to filamentous actin (F-actin) in type 1 autoimmune hepatitis.
Journal of clinical pathology, 2006. **59**(3): p. 280-284.
74. Clemente, M., et al, Enterocyte actin autoantibody detection: a new diagnostic tool in celiac disease diagnosis: results of a multicenter study. The American journal of gastroenterology, 2004. **99**(8): p. 1551-1556.
75. Marciano, F., M. Savoia, and P. Vajro, Celiac disease-related hepatic injury: Insights into associated conditions and underlying pathomechanisms. Digestive and Liver Disease, 2016. **48**(2): p. 112-119.
76. Ginés, P., et al, European Association for the Study of the Liver. EASL clinical practice guidelines on the management of ascites, spontaneous bacterial peritonitis, and hepatorenal syndrome in cirrhosis. J Hepatol, 2010. **53**(3).
77. Novacek, G., et al, Prevalence and clinical importance of hypertransaminasaemia in coeliac disease. European journal of gastroenterology & hepatology, 1999. **11**(3): p. 283-288.
78. Di Biase, A., et al, Autoimmune liver diseases in a paediatric population with coeliac disease- a 10-year single-centre experience. Alimentary pharmacology & therapeutics, 2010. **31**(2): p. 253-260.
79. van Gerven, N.M., et al, Seroprevalence of celiac disease in patients with autoimmune hepatitis. European journal of gastroenterology & hepatology, 2014. **26**(10): p. 1104-1107.
80. Vajro, P., et al, Pediatric celiac disease, cryptogenic hypertransaminasemia, and autoimmune hepatitis. Journal of pediatric gastroenterology and nutrition, 2013. **56**(6): p. 663-670.
81. Nastasio, S., et al, Celiac disease-associated autoimmune hepatitis in childhood: long-term response to treatment. Journal of pediatric gastroenterology and nutrition, 2013. **56**(6): p. 671-674.
82. Colecchia, A., et al, Coeliac disease and autoimmune hepatitis: Gluten-free diet can influence liver disease outcome. Digestive and Liver Disease, 2011. **43**(3): p. 247.
83. Lundin, K.E. and C. Wijmenga, Coeliac disease and autoimmune disease [mdash] genetic overlap and screening. Nature Reviews Gastroenterology & Hepatology, 2015. **12**(9): p. 507- 515.

84. Mirzaagha, F., et al, Coeliac disease in autoimmune liver disease: a cross-sectional study and a systematic review. Digestive and Liver Disease, 2010. **42**(9): p. 620-623.

85. Bridoux-Henno, L., et al, A case of celiac disease presenting with autoimmune hepatitis and erythroblastopenia. Journal of pediatric gastroenterology and nutrition, 2001. **33**(5): p. 616- 619.

86. Arvola, T., et al, Celiac disease, thyrotoxicosis, and autoimmune hepatitis in a child. Journal of pediatric gastroenterology and nutrition, 2002. **35**(1): p. 90-92.

87. Leonardi, S., et al, Autoimmune hepatitis associated with celiac disease in childhood: report of two cases. Journal of gastroenterology and hepatology, 2003. **18**(11): p. 1324-1327.

88. Biecker, E., et al, Autoimmune hepatitis, cryoglobulinaemia and untreated coeliac disease: a case report. European journal of gastroenterology & hepatology, 2003. **15**(4): p. 423-427.

89. Iorio, R., et al, Lack of benefit of gluten-free diet on autoimmune hepatitis in a boy with celiac disease. Journal of pediatric gastroenterology and nutrition, 2004. **39**(2): p. 207-210.

90. Tagle, M., et al, Coexistence of Celiac Disease and autoimmune hepatitis case study and literature review. Revista de gastroenterologia del Peru: organo oficial de la Sociedad de Gastroenterologia del Peru, 2006. **26**(1): p. 80.

91. Csak, T., et al, Holmes-Adie syndrome, autoimmune hepatitis and celiac disease: a case report. World Journal of Gastroenterology: WJG, 2006. **12**(9): p. 1485.

92. Ferrò, M.T., et al, A case of multiple sclerosis with atypical onset associated with autoimmune hepatitis and silent coeliac disease. Neurological Sciences, 2008. **29**(1): p. 29-31.

93. Ozaslan, E., Autoimmune hepatitis-autoimmune cholangitis overlap syndrome and autoimmune thyroiditis in a patient with celiac disease. European journal of gastroenterology & hepatology, 2009. **21**(6): p. 716-718.

94. Quail, M.A., et al, Seronegative autoimmune hepatitis presenting after diagnosis of coeliac disease: a case report. European journal of gastroenterology & hepatology, 2009. **21**(5): p. 576-579.

95. Tovoli, F., et al, Autoimmune hepatitis and celiac disease: case report showing an entero- hepatic link. Case reports in gastroenterology, 2010. **4**(3): p. 469-475.

96. Volta, U., et al, Fulminant type 1 autoimmune hepatitis in a recently diagnosed celiac disease patient. Archives of Iranian medicine, 2013. **16**(11): p.

683.

97. Dieli-Crimi, R., et al, An autoimmune polyglandular syndrome complicated with celiac disease and autoimmune hepatitis. Ann Hepatol, 2016. **15**: p. 588-591.

98. Iacono, O.L., et al, Anti-tissue transglutaminase antibodies in patients with abnormal liver tests: is it always coeliac disease? The American journal of gastroenterology, 2005. **100**(11):
p. 2472-2477.

99. Volta, U., et al, Coeliac disease hidden by cryptogenic hypertransaminasaemia. The Lancet, 1998. **352**(9121): p. 26-29.

100. Bardella, M.T., et al, Chronic unexplained hypertransaminasemia may be caused by occult celiac disease. Hepatology, 1999. **29**(3): p. 654-657.

101. Zanini, B., et al, Factors that contribute to hypertransaminasemia in patients with celiac disease or functional gastrointestinal syndromes. Clinical Gastroenterology and Hepatology, 2014. **12**(5): p. 804-810. e2.

102. Hatanaka, S.A., et al, The effect of a gluten-free diet on alanine aminotransferase (ALT) in celiac patients. Revista Colombiana de Gastroenterologia, 2015. **30**(4): p. 412-418.

103. Hagander, B., et al, Hepatic injury in adult coeliac disease. The lancet, 1977. **310**(8032): p. 270-272.

104. Jacobsen, M., et al, Hepatic lesions in adult coeliac disease. Scandinavian journal of gastroenterology, 1990. **25**(7): p. 656-662.

105. Bardella, M.T., et al, Prevalence of hypertransaminasemia in adult celiac patients and effect of gluten-free diet. Hepatology, 1995. **22**(3): p. 833-836.

106. Dickey, W., et al, Liver Abnormalities Associated with Celiac Sprue: How Common Are They, What Is Their Significance, and What Do We Do About Them? Journal of clinical gastroenterology, 1995. **20**(4): p. 290-292.

107. Foley, A., S. Shepherd, and P. Gibson, Frequency of elevated ALT in untreated coeliac disease and the impact of compliance with gluten free diet on ALT normalisation. Journal of Gastroenterology and Hepatology, 2009. **24**: p. A337.

108. Lewis, N., et al. PREVALENCE AND CONSEQUENCE OF HYPERTRANSAMINASAEMIA IN INCIDENT COELIAC DISEASE: HOW COMMON IS IT AND DOES IT MATTER? in Gut. 2009. BMJ PUBLISHING GROUP BRITISH MED ASSOC HOUSE, TAVISTOCK SQUARE, LONDON WC1H 9JR, ENGLAND.

109. Korpimäki, S., et al, Gluten-sensitive hypertransaminasemia in celiac disease: an infrequent and often subclinical finding. The American journal of

gastroenterology, 2011. **106**(9): p. 1689-1696.

110. Bonamico, M., et al, Hepatic damage in celiac disease in children. Minerva pediatrica, 1986.**38**(21): p. 959-962.

111. Farre, C., et al, Hypertransaminasemia in pediatric celiac disease patients and its prevalence as a diagnostic clue. The American journal of gastroenterology, 2002. **97**(12): p. 3176-3181.

112. Arslan, N., et al, The prevalence of liver function abnormalities in pediatric celiac disease patients and its relation with intestinal biopsy findings. Acta gastro-enterologica Belgica, 2005. **68**(4): p. 424-427.

113. Younossi, Z.M., et al, Global epidemiology of nonalcoholic fatty liver disease-Meta-analytic assessment of prevalence, incidence, and outcomes. Hepatology, 2016. **64**(1): p. 73-84.

114. Younossi, Z.M., et al, The economic and clinical burden of nonalcoholic fatty liver disease in the United States and Europe. Hepatology, 2016. **64**(5): p. 1577-1586.

115. Reilly, N.R., et al, Increased risk of non-alcoholic fatty liver disease after diagnosis of celiac disease. Journal of hepatology, 2015. **62**(6): p. 1405-1411.

116. Bardella, M., et al, Searching for coeliac disease in patients with non-alcoholic fatty liver disease. Digestive and Liver Disease, 2004. **36**(5): p. 333-336.

117. Bakhshipour, A., et al, Prevalence of coeliac disease in patients with non-alcoholic fatty liver disease. Arab Journal of Gastroenterology, 2013. **14**(3): p. 113-115.

118. Abenavoli, L., et al, Liver steatosis in celiac disease: the open door. Minerva gastroenterologica e dietologica, 2013. **59**(1): p. 89-95.

119. Abenavoli, L., et al, A pathogenetic link between non-alcoholic fatty liver disease and celiac disease. Endocrine, 2013. **43**(1): p. 65-67.

120. Narciso-Schiavon, J.L. and L. de Lucca Schiavon, Autoantibodies in chronic hepatitis C: A clinical perspective. World journal of hepatology, 2015. **7**(8): p. 1074.

121. Durante-Mangoni, E., et al, Silent celiac disease in chronic hepatitis C: impact of interferon treatment on the disease onset and clinical outcome. Journal of clinical gastroenterology, 2004. **38**(10): p. 901-905.

122. Thevenot, T., et al, Coeliac disease in chronic hepatitis C: a French multicentre prospective study. Alimentary pharmacology & therapeutics, 2007. **26**(9): p. 1209-1216.

123. Lim, E. and K. Watson, Unmasking of coeliac disease on interferon treatment for hepatitis C.

Internal medicine journal, 2010. **40**(1): p. 85-87.

124. Adinolfi, L.E., E.D. Mangoni, and A. Andreana, Interferon and ribavirin treatment for chronic hepatitis C may activate celiac disease. The American journal of gastroenterology, 2001. **96**(2): p. 607.

125. Leonardi, S. and M. La Rosa, Are hepatitis B virus and celiac disease linked? Hepatitis monthly, 2010. **10**(3): p. 173.

126. Sima, H., et al, The prevalence of celiac autoantibodies in hepatitis patients. Iranian Journal of Allergy, Asthma and Immunology, 2010. **9**(3): p. 157.

127. Heshin-Bekenstein, M., et al, Hepatitis B Virus Revaccination With Standard Versus Pre-S Vaccine in Previously Immunized Patients With Celiac Disease. Journal of pediatric gastroenterology and nutrition, 2015. **61**(4): p. 400-403.

128. Sharma, B.C., D.K. Bhasin, and R. Nada, Association of celiac disease with non-cirrhotic portal fibrosis. Journal of gastroenterology and hepatology, 2006. **21**(1): p. 332-334.

129. Singh, B., et al, Association of celiac disease and portal hypertension: Cirrhotic or noncirrhotic. Indian Journal of Gastroenterology, 2015. **34**(1): p. 77-77.

130. Musumba, C.O., et al, Acute variceal bleeding in a man with coeliac disease. Gut, 2013. **62**(5): p. 740-740.

131. Yazdani, S. and A. Abdizadeh, Coeliac disease as a potential cause of idiopathic portal hypertension: a case report. Gastroenterology report, 2016: p. gov065.

132. Maiwall, R., et al, Investigation into celiac disease in Indian patients with portal hypertension. Indian Journal of Gastroenterology, 2014. **33**(6): p. 517-523.

133. Eapen, C., et al, Non-cirrhotic intrahepatic portal hypertension: associated gut diseases and prognostic factors. Digestive diseases and sciences, 2011. **56**(1): p. 227-235.

134. Ferrari, F., M. Mennini, and S. Cucchiara, Portal hypertension and celiac disease: A true association? Indian Journal of Gastroenterology, 2015. **34**(3): p. 273-274.

135. Duman, A.E., et al, Cirrhosis and intestinal B-cell lymphoma: two entities that are rarely associated with celiac disease. The Turkish journal of gastroenterology: the official journal of Turkish Society of Gastroenterology, 2013. **24**(2): p. 192-194.

136. Demir, H., et al, Cirrhosis in children with celiac disease. Journal of clinical gastroenterology, 2005. **39**(7): p. 630-633.

137. Dekaken, A., et al, Cirrhosis revealing silent celiac disease: a case report. Immunoanalysis & Specialised Biology, 2013. **28**(2): p. 137-139.

138. Ratziu, V., M. Nourani, and T. Poynard, Discussion on celiac disease in patients with severe liver disease: gluten-free diet may reverse hepatic failure. Gastroenterology, 2002. **123**(6): p. 2158-2159.

139. Roumeliotis, N., M. Hosking, and O. Guttman, Celiac disease and cardiomyopathy in an adolescent with occult cirrhosis. Paediatrics & child health, 2012. **17**(8): p. 437-439.

140. Pavone, P., et al, Liver transplantation in a child with celiac disease. Journal of gastroenterology and hepatology, 2005. **20**(6): p. 956-960.

141. Casswall, T.H., et al, Severe liver damage associated with celiac disease: findings in six toddler-aged girls. European journal of gastroenterology & hepatology, 2009. **21**(4): p. 362- 369.

142. Cotter, M.B., et al, Coeliac-like duodenal pathology in orthotopic liver transplant patients on mycophenolic acid therapy. Histopathology, 2015. **66**(4): p. 500-507.

143. <celiac-disease Fmc- HGE 2013.pdf>.

# APPENDIX

## Appendix 1: Prevalence of CD in cirrhosis and effect of RSG on liver function

| Name | | Alcohol (Ethyl index) | |
|---|---|---|---|
| Age | | Profession | |
| Gender | | Socio economic | |
| ND | | Level of study | |
| Tobacco (PA) | | Lifestyle | |

| ATCD Fx : MC : | | yes | no |
|---|---|---|---|
| Chronic liver disease : | | yes | no |
| Cirrhosis : | | yes | no |
| CHC : | | yes | no |
| Immune deficiency : | | yes | no |

P: dysimmune disease :

Insulin-dependent diabetes: yes no

Thyroiditis: yes no If yes: aetiology :

## Treatment :

| Psoriasis : | yes | no |
|---|---|---|
| vitiligo : | yes | no |
| Ataxia  : | yes | no |
| Trisomy 21 : | yes | no |
| Dermatitis herpetiformis : | yes | no |
| CBP : | yes | no |

Other: hypertension / type 2 diabetes / dyslipidaemia / SAD

**FRH** :dental care / Scarification

Tattoo/unprotected sex Surgery/transfusion
**Data relating to Cirrhosis :**

Revealing mode :

Development time :

Clinical and biological data

## Clinic

| | |
|---|---|
| Stellate angioma : | HMG : |
| Palmar erythrosis : | Ascites : |
| Atrophy of eminence Tenar and hypothenar : | HVAC : |
| Digital hippocratism : | SMG : |
| Gynecomastia : | IMO : |
| Biology | |
| GB : | B viral serology : |
| Hb : | Viral serology C : |
| Plaq : | AAN : |
| ASAT : | Anti-LKM1 : |
| ALAT : | Ac anti mitochondria : |
| PA : | Ac anti-smooth muscle : |
| GGT : | Ig A : |
| BT : | IgG : |
| Albumin : | IgM : |
| TP : | Cupraemia |
| INR : | Cupriuria |
| Creatinemia : | Ceruloplasmin |
| Blood glucose : | $\alpha_1$ antitrypsin |
| Cholesterol : | Serum serum |
| Triglyceride : | CST |

# Morphological data :

| FOGD | Ultrasound |
|---|---|
| VO : | Dysmorphic liver |
| VG | SMG |
| IGV | HVAC |
| GOV | Ascites |
| GHT | Thrombosis VSH |
| Aspect of the duodenum :<br>-crenellated appearance of the duodenal folds<br>-reduction in the height of folds<br>-rarefaction of the duodenal folds<br>-Mosaic appearance<br>-erosive duodenitis<br>-ulcerated duodenitis | Portal thrombosis |
| Etiology | Etiological treatment |
| Viral hepatitis B | Antiviral treatment: D-Penicillamine: Azathioprine : ursodeoxycholic acid : |
| Viral hepatitis C | |
| HAI | |
| CBP | |
| CSP | |
| Hepatic steatosis | |
| Haemochromatosis | |
| Granulomatous hepatitis | |
| Cryptogenic : | |

## Child-pugh stage:MELD :

# Complications :

| Type | Number of episodes | treatment | evolution |
|---|---|---|---|
| DOA | | | |
| Refractory ascites | | | |
| Digestive haemorrhage | | | |
| ISLA | | | |
| Hepatic encephalopathy | | | |
| Hydrothorax | | | |

**Data relating to celiac disease: Positive diagnosis :**
Serology: anti-transglutaminase Ac: anti-EMA Ac :
Duodenal biops
Marsh stage:.
DMO :

**RSG:** Compliance: Duration of follow-up: **Impact on :**

| General condition | |
|---|---|
| Weight | |
| Hb | |
| albuminemia | |
| ferritinemia | |
| bilirubin | |
| ALAT | |
| ASAT | |
| PA | |
| GGT | |
| TP | |
| INR | |
| VO | |
| Ascites | |
| Child score | |
| MELD score | |
| Celiac serology | |
| Histology (duodenal biopsy) | |
| Liver histology if performed | |

**Follow-up period :**

# Appendix 2: Child pugh score

|  | 1 point | 2 points | 3 points |
|---|---|---|---|
| Ascites | absent | moderate | Tense or refractory to diuretics |
| Bilirubin ( µmol/l) | <35 | 35-50 | >50 |
| Albumin (g/l) | >35 | 28-35 | <28 |
| INR TP | <1,7 >50% | 1,7 -2,2 40-50% | >2,2 <40% |
| Encephalopathy | Absent | Mild to moderate (stage 1-2) | Severe (stage 3-4) |
| The prognosis for cirrhosis is based on the total score of : Child -pugh A (5-6 points): 100% survival to 1 year Child -pughB( 7 - 9 points): 80% survival to 1 year Child -pughC( 10-15 points): 45% survival to 1 year | | | |

# Appendix 3: MELD score

| Frequency of use | | |
|---|---|---|
| Liver transplantation | MELD>15: benefit of transplantation, the MELD determines the order of priority on the waiting list, with a few exceptions (HCC). | +++ |
| Selection of patients for TIPS placement | MELD<8: good prognosis MELD>18: poorer prognosis MELD>24: prohibitive mortality | ++ |
| Alcoholic hepatitis | Prediction of risk of 90-day mortality MELD>18: indication for corticosteroid therapy in the absence of contraindications (retrospective studies) | ++ |
| Major surgery (digestive, orthopaedic or other) cardiac) | Mortality risk prediction at 1 week, 1 month, 3 months, 1 year and 5 years | ++ |
| Type II hepatorenal syndrome | MELD<20: median survival 11 months MELD>=20 :median survival 3 months | + |
| Cirrhosis with sepsis unrelated to PBS | MELD was described as the only significant factor predicting mortality in this situation. MELD<20: 3-month survival >90%. | + |

MELD>=20: 3-month survival:60%.

The formula for calculating the score is as follows: 3.8 x loge (Bb [mg/dl]) + 11.2 x loge (INR) + 9.6 x loge (creatinine [mg/dl]) + 6.4 x (cause of cirrhosis: 0 if cholestasis or alcoholic, 1 in other cases)].

# Appendix 4: Marsh's modified classification of gluten-induced small bowel lesions

| | |
|---|---|
| Stage 0 | Pre-infiltrated mucosa; up to 30% of patients with dermatitis herpetiformis (DH) or with gluten-related ataxia have apparently normal small intestine biopsies |
| Stage 1 | Increase in the number of intraepithelial lymphocytes (IEL) to over 30 per 100 enterocytes |
| Stage 2 | Crypt hyperplasia. In addition to the increase in LELs, the depth of the crypts is increased without any reduction in the height of the villi. These changes may be induced by a gluten challenge, but may also be present in 20% of patients with a gluten deficiency. untreated patients with dermatitis herpetiformis and celiac disease |
| Stage 3 | Villous atrophy: A, partial; B, subtotal; C, total. This stage corresponds to the so-called classic aspect of coeliac disease and is observed in 40% of patients with DH. Despite pronounced changes in the mucosa, many individuals are asymptomatic and therefore classified as sub-clinical or silent cases. This lesion, although characteristic, is not sufficient to diagnose coeliac disease, as it is also found in cases of severe lambliasis, food allergy in children, graft-versus-host disease, chronic ischaemia of the small intestine, tropical sprue, immunoglobulin deficiency and other diseases. and graft rejection |

# Appendix 5: Diagnostic algorithm for celiac disease (adapted from [143]

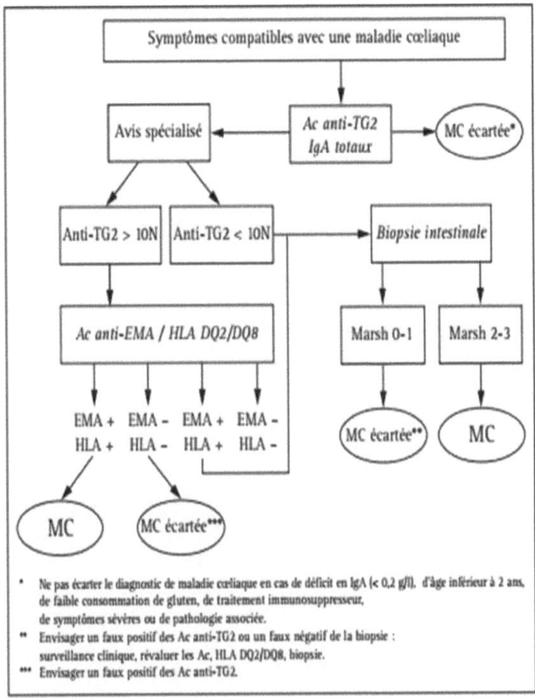

# TABLE OF CONTENTS

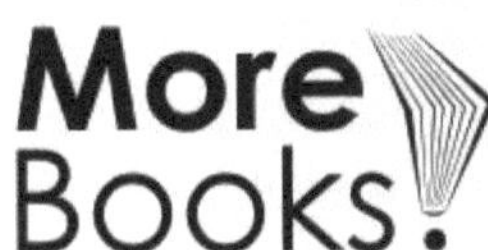



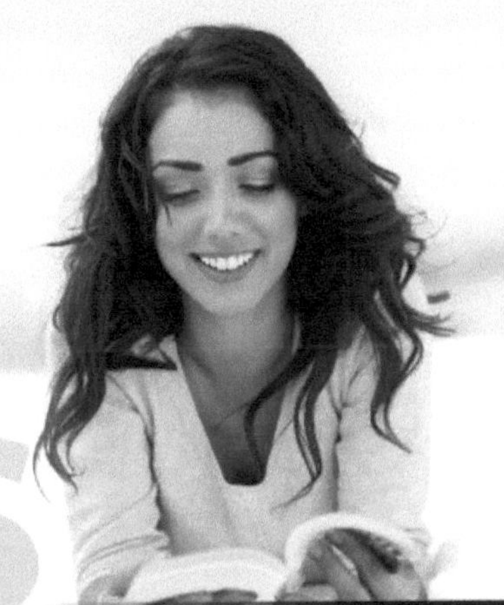

# yes

# I want morebooks!

Buy your books fast and straightforward online - at one of world's fastest growing online book stores! Environmentally sound due to Print-on-Demand technologies.

Buy your books online at
**www.morebooks.shop**

Kaufen Sie Ihre Bücher schnell und unkompliziert online – auf einer der am schnellsten wachsenden Buchhandelsplattformen weltweit! Dank Print-On-Demand umwelt- und ressourcenschonend produziert.

Bücher schneller online kaufen
**www.morebooks.shop**

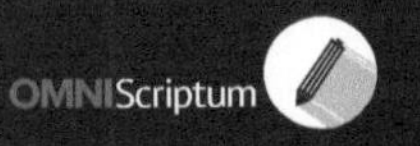

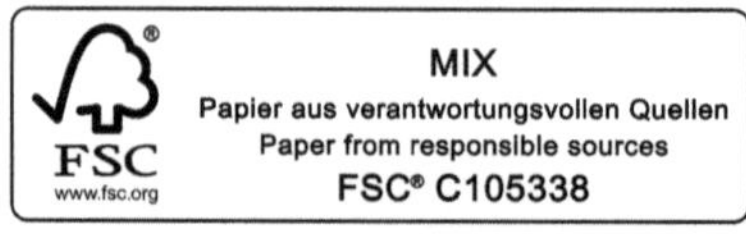

Printed by Books on Demand GmbH, Norderstedt / Germany